Caring for a Living

International Policy Exchange Series

Published in collaboration with the
Center for International Policy Exchanges
University of Maryland

Series Editors

Douglas J. Besharov
Neil Gilbert

United in Diversity?
Comparing Social Models in Europe and America
Edited by Jens Alber and Neil Gilbert

The Korean State and Social Policy:
How South Korea Lifted Itself from Poverty and Dictatorship to Affluence and Democracy
Stein Ringen, Huck-ju Kwon, Ilcheong Yi, Taekyoon Kim, and Jooha Lee

Child Protection Systems:
International Trends and Orientations
Edited by Neil Gilbert, Nigel Parton, and Marit Skivenes

The Age of Dualization:
The Changing Face of Inequality in Deindustrializing Societies
Edited by Patrick Emmenegger, Silja Häusermann, Bruno Palier, and Martin Seeleib-Kaiser

Counting the Poor:
New Thinking About European Poverty Measures and Lessons for the United States
Edited by Douglas J. Besharov and Kenneth A. Couch

Social Policy and Citizenship:
The Changing Landscape
Edited by Adalbert Evers and Anne-Marie Guillemard

Chinese Policy in a Time of Transition
Edited by Douglas J. Besharov and Karen Baehler

Reconciling Work and Poverty Reduction:
How Successful Are European Welfare States?
Edited by Bea Cantillon and Frank Vandenbroucke

University Adaptation in Difficult Economic Times
Edited by Paola Mattei

Workfare Revisited:
Activation or Workfare? Governance and the Neo-Liberal Convergence
Edited by Ivar Lødemel and Amílcar Moreira

Child Welfare Systems and Migrant Children:
A Cross Country Study of Policies and Practice in Children
Edited by Marit Skivenes, Ravinder Barn, Katrin Kriz, and Tarja Pösö

Adjusting to a World in Motion:
Trends in Global Migration and Migration Policy
Edited by Douglas J. Besharov and Mark H. Lopez

Caring for a Living:
Migrant Women, Aging Citizens, and Italian Families
Francesca Degiuli

UNIVERSITY OF MARYLAND 1856

SCHOOL of
PUBLIC POLICY

CARING FOR A LIVING

Migrant Women, Aging Citizens, and Italian Families

FRANCESCA DEGIULI

OXFORD
UNIVERSITY PRESS

OXFORD
UNIVERSITY PRESS

Oxford University Press is a department of the University of Oxford. It furthers the University's objective of excellence in research, scholarship, and education by publishing worldwide.Oxford is a registered trade mark of Oxford University Press in the UK and certain other countries.

Published in the United States of America by Oxford University Press
198 Madison Avenue, New York, NY 10016, United States of America.

Library of Congress Cataloging-in-Publication Data
Names: Degiuli, Francesca, author.
Title: Caring for a living : migrant women, aging citizens, and Italian families / Francesca Degiuli.
Description: Oxford ; New York : Oxford University Press, [2016] | Series: International policy exchange series | Includes bibliographical References and index.
Identifiers: LCCN 2015041097 | ISBN 9780199989010 (alk. paper)
Subjects: LCSH: Older people—Care—Italy. | Long-term care of the sick—Italy. | Caregivers—Italy. | Women foreign workers—Italy.
Classification: LCC HV1454.2.I8 D44 2016 | DDC 362.6/30945—dc23
LC record available at http://lccn.loc.gov/2015041097

9 8 7 6 5 4 3 2 1
Printed by Sheridan, USA

I dedicate this book to my mother, Maria Luisa Fassino, who was always very supportive of my choices, even when they were difficult for her to accept. Thank you for all the love you have given me from the day I was born to the last day of your life. It was an incredible gift.

CONTENTS

ACKNOWLEDGMENTS

This book is the result of a great personal and intellectual journey that has expanded over a long stretch of time and space and because of that I need to include in thoughts of gratitude a very large number of people to whom I am deeply indebted.

My first acknowledgments go to the women, and the few men, whose lives provide the basis for this project. I would like to thank them for sharing their stories, their minds, their families, and their time with me. I wish to thank them for their trust, generosity, patience, and great insights, not only on home eldercare work and migration but on matters of life more in general. In addition, I want to express my deepest gratitude to Dalisay and Corina for helping me get through the last months of my mother's life. Without your invaluable help I would not have been able to manage being a mother, a daughter, and a researcher at the same time. Thank you.

I also want to express my most heartfelt gratitude to all the women of Tierra for their kindness and willingness to answer my many questions and for sharing many delicious meals at the center. In particular I want to thank the Carework Group for their friendship, the stimulating conversations, the great research opportunities, and the many good dinners they offered me during both of my stays in Torino.

A heartfelt thanks also goes to my mentors at the University of California, Santa Barbara who have helped me to design, start, and bring to completion a first draft of this project as my doctoral dissertation. Thank you KumKum Bhavnani and Rich Appelbaum for the many hours you spent with me talking about this project, for your enthusiasm, your support, your insights and comments, and your careful reading of the first draft of this manuscript. Thanks also to John Foran for his careful reading of this project and for providing many words of kindness and encouragement throughout my graduate years. I am also very grateful to Grace Chang, not only for providing me with a framework to think about women and domestic work beyond the confines of the home and of national boundaries, but also for gently pushing me to find more nuanced and complex answers when exploring the complex relationships between women. Many thanks also to Eileen Boris for her encouragement and support throughout the completion of my dissertation and beyond, and the many engaging conversations on the issue of home care both in the United States and in Italy.

A special thanks goes also to my many different writing groups that, throughout the years and in different locations, have helped me to bring this project to completion. Without them this project would never have taken its current shape. I would like to thank Karl Bryant, Hillary Haldane, Helene Lee, and Mark Shuller for their insightful comments, friendship, laughter, and emotional support while writing the first draft of this book and Rafael de la Dehesa, Hosu Kim, and Jean Halley for the invaluable help they have provided throughout the completion of this manuscript in the form of comments, edits, discussion, friendship, and, of course, food. I am very grateful for your "being there" for me and for literally getting me through the arduous process of writing. A special thanks also goes to my former colleague Kate Crehan who helped me get through a difficult patch near the end of the book with her careful and beautifully phrased comments. And, of course, many, many thanks to Chris Kapp and Terry Haywoode for their copyediting skills. Thanks for greatly improving the readability of this manuscript.

Thank you also to the many CUNY colleagues who in different ways and in different capacities have contributed to this project, among them Maria Rice Bellamy, Bilge Yesil, Siona Wilson, Namita Manohar, Kelly Secovnie, Marcela Echeverri, Stephanie Rupp, Jay Arena, Tom Volscho, Ananya Mukherjea, and Ismael Garcia Colon.

A special mention among my former colleagues also goes to Leigh Bingham for bringing me back to this project when I was getting pulled in different research directions and to Roz Bologh for her kindness and constant support throughout the years.

Thanks also to the University of California, Santa Barbara for providing me with the seed money to start this research project, to CUNY for providing funds to continue this project, and to Fairleigh Dickinson University for the research release time that allowed me to complete this manuscript. I would also like to thank the Center for European and Mediterranean Studies at New York University for granting me a visiting fellowship that in the past couple of years has allowed me to meet engaging and stimulating colleagues and to participate in enriching debates and programs.

I would also like to express my gratitude to my current colleagues in the department of History and Social Sciences for making me feel at home among them, for challenging me to bring an interdisciplinary lens to my project, and for helping me to maintain a good balance between teaching, researching, and writing.

A special mention goes also to the editors at Oxford University Press who have been advocates for this project: thanks to Nicolas Liu, Dana Bliss, and Andrew Dominello for your support, guidance, and assistance at different stages in the manuscript review and publication preparation process. A thankful thought also goes to the anonymous reviewers who have offered informed and constructive critiques that have helped to move my project forward. And, finally, thank you also to Devasena Vedamurthi and her team for making the project ready for production.

I am also very grateful for all my friends and family here in the United States and in Italy for being there for me at different stages of this project, for being who you are, for feeding me, for making me laugh, for arguing with me, and for being a great part of my life. It would be too long to list you all but be aware that I have all of you in my mind while I write these few lines. I need, however, to express my deepest gratitude to my friend and fellow sociologist Helene Lee for being the greatest pal even in the most stressful times of my life. Thank you.

Last, but not least, I would like to acknowledge and thank my fabulous daughters Bianca and Giada for filling my life with love, for telling me when it is time to stop working and start playing, and for making life in general more interesting and worth living. My last thought goes to my husband and partner in crime Andrew Cammarano for being there throughout all the different phases of this project in different capacities. I deeply thank you for your love, friendship, and moral and material support throughout this journey. I greatly owe you.

INTRODUCTION

One afternoon, while sitting with a cup of coffee in a kitchen full of light, in the apartment I had recently rented from her in Turin, Italy, Maurizia, an Italian woman in her mid-60s, aware of my research interests, told me:

> My mother has always been depressed, she was already taking medications for it, but at some point in her late 60s things began to worsen. She had two serious episodes, two major hysterical crises, so extreme that we had to take her to the ER. The psychiatrist on call the second time we took her told us that he wasn't sure but that it looked like the beginning of dementia, senile dementia that is, and in the end he was right. In the beginning the process was gradual but then it started to progress faster. She lost the language, she is now often confused, she wakes up in the middle of the night not knowing where she is or who she is... Today she needs assistance 24 hours a day, seven days a week... At the beginning I was able to manage it. I lived up here, she lived in the apartment below... it was do-able... but when things got worse I was no longer able to manage and neither could my brother... I have a job, a daughter, a partner... so we decided to look for somebody. We asked around, we tried an Italian first, an older woman, a widow, but my mother did not like her, then a colleague of mine who had a badante from Moldova told me about this girl.... When she came here the first time she barely spoke Italian so I was going to hire somebody else, a Peruvian who already had some experience and spoke Italian, but then the Peruvian had a car accident so... Irina it

> was. She has been living with my mother ever since... I come often, as you can see, three to four times a week but Irina manages well.

A few months later, once again sitting in front of a cup of coffee in the kitchen located directly below mine, a kitchen in which time seemed to have stopped 10 years ago, Irina, after having observed my family and me during our comings and going in the building for a while and after many occasional encounters on the balcony hanging clothes, knowing my interest in her work, decided to share her experience. She told me:

> I came to Italy from Moldova in 2000 when the economy there was collapsing. I made that decision because the hospital where I was working as a head nurse stopped paying our salaries. I decided to come to Italy for a year, to make some money and then go back. My husband tried first, but he could not find anything. For women, it is easier.... When I got here I did not speak the language. I went to work for another family for two weeks, to help a friend, but then I met Maurizia and Alessia. They took me in and they became my family. Their house became my house. I take care of everything here but above all I take care of Alessia. My workday starts at around 7 a.m. when my daughters, who live with us, at the moment, wake up and get ready to go to school; they do everything on their own while I, on the other hand, make myself a cup of coffee and get mentally ready for the day. Then I look around and figure out what needs to be done in the house. I may start lunch or I do laundry... it depends. At around 9:30 a.m. I wake nonna[1] up, I help her to get up and go to the bathroom. There I wash her, I comb her, and then we go back to the bedroom to put on a dress, sometimes also some make up, then I make her breakfast and give her the medications. After breakfast we sit down and we look at some books together, or I try to explain to her what is on television. I try to keep her mind engaged, to make her work, but it's not always easy. Sometimes she gets agitated, she gets confused and scared and I need to comfort her. When that happens I can't do anything else, I have to focus on her, make her talk, bring her back... If she's good and comfortable instead I have more time to do other chores. Then I prepare lunch, we eat, I clean dishes, then I clean her. This is when she goes to bed for a nap. That's when I have some time to myself, usually it lasts more or less an hour, and then it starts all over again, for seven days a week, twenty-four hours a day.

The experiences Maurizia and Irina shared with me, in the quiet space of private apartments in Torino, aside from describing a specific instance, provide us with a glimpse of new labor relationships that are becoming more common in many postindustrial societies in which the need for long-term eldercare is growing and where im/migrant[2] women increasingly fill this void. The world of today is aging and is doing so at a great speed. According to the United Nations the global share of people 60 years and over increased from 9.2% in 1990 to 11.7% in 2013 and will continue to grow, reaching 21.1% by 2050. In addition, by 2047 this sector of the population is expected to exceed that of children, dramatically inverting the age balance of the world population for the first time in history. These remarkable changes are, for the most part, the result of a global drop in fertility but also of new technological and medical developments that have helped to extend the life expectancy of many, particularly in the wealthy countries of the Global North (United Nations Department of Economic and Social Affairs, 2013). Today people are living longer and this certainly represents one of the greatest achievements of the past century; however, this development comes with its own problems, one of them being an increased need for long-term care. Aging populations, even when healthy, require a higher degree of care and support in accomplishing daily activities due to progressive functional and cognitive limitations. This is a need that increases steeply when multiple chronic conditions and more complex pathologies such as senile dementia, Alzheimer's disease, and Parkinson's disease are added to the natural progression of aging, a development that becomes particularly common among the oldest old (80 years and over). The U.S. government, for example, estimates that 70% of the population 65 years and older will most likely require some form of long-term care during their lifetime (US Department of Health and Human Services, 2015). Who is going to provide this care and in what form is a question currently haunting many high-income and middle-income countries, but it will soon be shared by most of the world. This growing demand for care comes at a time when families, and particularly women, are already struggling to fulfill all of the care needed for social reproduction. Contemporary processes such as increased women's participation in the labor force, the progressive deconstruction of extended and even nuclear families, and growing labor mobility have left a great number of societies with what Arlie Hochschild (1997) has defined as a "care deficit." This deficit is worsened by the fact that welfare states, instead of stepping in to support struggling families, are increasingly retrenching in order to reduce their costs, while at the same time pushing care work out of hospitals and institutions and handing it back to families (Aronson & Neysmith, 1996; Ungerson, 2000).

To participate in this debate I chose to explore the organization and the provision of long-term care for the elderly in a country already in the midst of an eldercare crisis: Italy. With one of the oldest populations in the world, second to Japan and on par with Germany (ISTAT, 2014; World Bank, 2015), a long-standing negative growth rate, decreasing numbers of available unpaid caregivers, and an inadequate state response to address these demographic developments, the country provides an important case study in understanding the difficulties generated by the growing need for long-term eldercare. The Italian response to a growing deficit in eldercare has taken the shape of *home eldercare assistance*, an arrangement whereby long-term care services are bought in the market in the form of private and individualized assistance by families sometimes with the help of cash provisions provided by the state. The providers of these services, which range from live-in jobs requiring 24/7 assistance to live-out ones requiring only a few hours a day, commonly known as *badanti*[3] (minders), are predominantly immigrant women,[4] less often men, coming from different areas of the world ranging from Peru to Moldova, from the Philippines to Somalia for whom the state has made special provisions in terms of immigration law.

Although Italy is not the only country to make use of im/migrant workers to fill the increasing demand for eldercare, a phenomenon widespread in most of Europe (among others, Cancedda, 2001; van Hooren, 2014) and to a lesser degree in many parts of Asia, North America, and Latin America (Lan, 2006; Vega Solis, 2009), in Italy this organization of care has become the predominant one, to the point that care scholars Bettio, Simonazzi, and Villa (2006, p. 272) describe the current Italian model of care no longer as a "family-centered" one but as a "migrant in the family" one.[5] While it is difficult to provide a definitive total concerning the number of workers employed as home eldercare assistants, due to the presence of a large contingent of irregular im/migrant workers in this job and the porous boundaries between domestic and eldercare, it is estimated that this occupation currently involves between 500,000 and 1,655,000 workers (Ambrosini, 2015: ISTAT, 2014) scattered across the territory, albeit with a greater concentration in North and Central Italy.[6] Aside from being widespread, home eldercare assistance has also proven to be a very resilient organization. From its inception in the mid-1990s to today, in fact, home eldercare assistance has grown in numbers, it has spread throughout the country, and it has become rooted in Italian society, notwithstanding the economic crisis of 2008–2009 and its aftermath, the austerity programs of recent years, and the growing difficulties that families experience in paying for care.

The goal of this book is to explore the emergence and the development of this new organization of care and the role that different social actors, including the state, Italian families, and the workers themselves, play in shaping and in defining it. To this day there are few qualitative studies that focus exclusively on home eldercare assistance and its provision (Da Roit, 2007; Sgritta, 2009; Stacey, 2011). Many of the studies concerned with the growing global transfer of care tend to concentrate on domestic work and treat eldercare only as a subset of that labor (Andall, 2000; Anderson, 2000; Boris & Parreñas, 2010; Chang, 2000; Ehrenreich & Hochschild, 2002; Gutiérrez Rodriguez, 2010; Hondagneu-Sotelo, 2001; Lan, 2006; Lutz, 2011; Parreñas, 2001; Sassen, 2001; Yeates, 2009), others instead focus only on specific national or racial/ethnic groups performing that labor (Ibarra, 2002; Vietti, 2012), whereas the growing number of social policy studies exploring the topic tend to be quantitative and to focus on welfare states and their comparisons (Cangiano, 2014; Da Roit & Weicht, 2013; van Hooren, 2014). This book instead centers on home eldercare assistance as an occupation of its own because, although short-term and long-term eldercare may include some elements of domestic work, the requirements of the job and the relationships between family caregivers, the workers, and the elders are qualitatively different. It does so by adopting a qualitative approach that makes it possible to place at the center of the inquiry the lived experiences of women, such as Maurizia and Irina, instead of the abstract concepts of *family* and *market*. This focus is important because it permits an exploration not only of what short-term and long-term eldercare entails for both the family caregivers and the im/migrant workers who provide it, but an exploration of the structure of the job, of who shapes it and how, of the discrepancies between what is deemed worthy of pay and what is not, of the relationships that emerge in these triangular relationships of labor, and of the ways in which gender and racial relations are produced, negotiated, and challenged among the workers, the employers, and the elders themselves.

To understand all of these different dimensions the book centers on the following questions: Who is expected to provide long-term care for the elders and in what form? What causes Italian families to hire im/migrant home eldercare assistants to provide this care? What does the job of a home eldercare assistant entail? How are im/migrant women from different backgrounds and levels of education channeled into *home eldercare assistance?* How does the state participate in shaping the relationship between families and im/migrant workers? How does the presence of an im/migrant home eldercare assistant change the gendered relations of care inside the home?

In the process of answering these questions the book engages several contemporary themes: first, it investigates the reasons behind the progressive aging of the population in most areas of the world, the increasing extension of the life span, particularly in wealthy countries, and the new needs for long-term care that these two developments combined generate. Second, it explores the demographic, economic, political, social, and cultural influences that have transformed the family unit and the gender roles within it, thereby changing its ability to provide care. Third, it analyzes the ways in which economic and political ideologies at the global level affect the shape of current welfare states and their relationships to families and markets. It also explores how these ideologies translate in the practice of the Italian welfare state and the consequences they determine. Fourth, it investigates the relationships between global, regional, and national processes that dislocate large pools of disposable feminized labor and the regional and national ones that instead control the relocation of these subjects. Fifth, it explores the many societal mechanisms that help to transform im/migrants coming from a wide variety of backgrounds in terms of nationalities, class, educational skills, and provenance into the unskilled labor force needed to provide home eldercare assistance in the current form. Sixth, it explores the ways in which employers use preconceived notions of culture, of race and ethnicity, and of nationalism to create the "ideal" employee and generate hierarchies of labor. These explorations taken together result in a better understanding of the specifics of the Italian case, and, in addition, offer valuable insights on long-term care and its provision that not only can inform future discussions on the matter but also, possibly, to envision new more equitable forms of eldercare.

Most importantly, investigations of these different links allow us to demystify the idea that the current organization of care is a simple market solution involving individual families in need of long-term care (*demand*) as well as im/migrant workers needing jobs (*supply*). The analysis shows that the creation of this specific market is the result of the convergence of complex and sometimes apparently contradictory global, regional, and national processes, shaped in their current form not only by economic ideas but also by cultural expectations, regional and national policies, global ideologies, and gendered norms. The result is a market that, in order to come into existence, relies on many levels of inequality and because of that is highly unstable, does not provide long-term solutions, and, in its current form, exposes two of society's most vulnerable subjects, the elderly and the im/migrant worker, to multiple levels of abuse.

Yet the presence of this market is essential because it allows the Italian state to avoid direct engagement with the problem. Although some scholars explain this lack of engagement through the notion of "institutional inertia" (Ranci & Sabatinelli, 2014), I argue that instead this lack of engagement allows the Italian state to fully become a neoliberal state. By simultaneously providing a program of cash for care with no strings attached and a segmented im/migrant labor force to provide basic eldercare needs to all social strata of the Italian population while helping them to maintain a fictional gendered status quo, the state progressively disengages itself from many of its former functions. It does so by taking advantage of its relatively strong position in the world system and in the process it reproduces and strengthens national, gendered, and racial inequalities.

CONTEXTUALIZING THE PROJECT

The questions addressed in this project were designed as a result of a constant interchange between my data and different literatures; two in particular have helped to shape the organization of this project: on the one hand the body of work exploring the global transfer of care and on the other, the literature on care and social policy.[7] The first is a literature that, starting at the beginning of this century, began to explore what scholars have defined as the "global nanny chain" (Hochschild, 2000) or as the "international division of reproductive labor" (Parreñas, 2001), a system of care in which the growing demand for care and domestic work in wealthy countries is filled by im/migrant women who often have to leave their children behind to be cared for by another domestic worker or a relative (among other Andall, 2000; Anderson, 2000; Boris & Parreñas, 2010; Chang, 2000; Ehrenreich & Hochschild, 2002; Gutiérrez-Rodriguez, 2010; Hondagneu-Sotelo, 2001; Lan, 2006; Lutz, 2011; Parreñas, 2001; Sassen, 2001; Yeates, 2009). The work of these scholars has been crucial in helping me frame the emergence and organization of home eldercare assistance in Italy not simply as the result of a national organization of care but also as the result of more complex processes started much further away. Their work, in fact, brought to the fore the connections between the increasing marketization of care in the Global North and processes of labor force dislocations in the Global South and in many countries of the former Soviet Union, processes that are increasingly feminized (Enloe, 1990, 2000; Freeman, 2000; Ibarra, 2002; Kofman et al., 2000; Mills, 1999; Ward, 2000; Zlotnik, 1995). These processes, among others, involved labor market transformations, the adoption of neoliberal policies in the form of structural adjustment programs, the progressive destruction of the commons and of former local communities, the progressive expansion of free market ideologies in every area of the world, and increasing wage inequality across countries. Understanding the macro and microlevel reasons behind the increasing presence of a feminized pool of workers is essential for the study of home eldercare because it provides important information on how workers will participate in the labor market. Migrants involved in circulatory migration have needs and expectations different from immigrants who are coming from distant regions of the world and who may have already accumulated a great deal of debt through migration. The same is true for workers who plan for temporary migratory journeys versus those who want to stay and integrate in the receiving societies. In addition, this literature helps to qualify and explain the many processes that often lie behind apparently voluntary migration projects.

Similarly, the examination of how these workers are incorporated into destination countries provides insights on the many societal processes, besides political and economic ones, that are involved in the creation, shaping and management of the immigrant workforce. Cultural, racial, and gendered understandings, in fact, are as crucial as laws and wages in defining and formalizing the way in which im/migrant workers are able to participate in the labor market. The perceptions of employers are very important for im/migrant workers who, for the most part, participate in informal relationships of labor. These perceptions influence how the workers are going to be treated, the relationships that they will be able to establish, and also the kinds of jobs that will become available to them and in what forms. Global and regional inequalities help to frame these workers in specific ways that inevitably influence their participation in the life of destination countries. In this sense the literature on the global transfer of care is, to this day, crucial in helping to explore how the inequalities existing at the global level, generated in many cases through colonization and currently exacerbated by global economic and political processes, are reproduced in the private relationships between employers and employees in the privacy of the home.

While it is widely recognized that this literature has played a very important role in elucidating the complex interplay between global and local processes in shaping the current organization of care, it has been criticized, especially early in its development, for downplaying the role of the state in shaping these relationships, for focusing too closely on care exclusively as a private relationship between families and workers and for ignoring many other dimensions, such as work in institutional settings, the variety of care (health, education, sexual), and the presence of men in the field, (Lutz, 2008; Mahon & Robinson, 2011; Williams, 2011; Yeates, 2009).

The criticism regarding the state, which I share, led me to turn to the care and social policy literature, a body of work that investigates the nature of state involvement in the organization of care. As care and social policy scholar Fiona Williams has pointed out, in Europe the new demands for care are not shaped simply by an absence of care provisions as they are, for example, in the United States, rather they are strongly influenced by contemporary changes in welfare provisions (Williams, 2011, pp. 22–23), existing migration policies, and the current shape of labor markets. The presence of the state in shaping the arrangement of care is reflected in my interviews, in which both unpaid family caregivers and im/migrant workers made it clear that their experiences were deeply defined and shaped both by the absence and the presence of it. Discussions of eldercare and eldercare choices often involved a discussion of the absence of state services for care, the absence of state-provided information on care, the choice of home eldercare assistance as the only available option, the bureaucracy of the welfare state, and the state in the form of cash allowances. Discussions with im/migrant workers, instead, involved the state in relation to immigration policies, work permits, amnesties, criminalization of migration, rigidity of the labor market and resistance in recognizing education and skills acquired in foreign countries. To fully understand the current arrangement of care it is therefore important to examine how the state operates at a mesolevel through policies regulating care, employment, and migration (Williams, 2012).

To better understand the relationship between the state and care provision I adopted the definition of care provided by Daly and Lewis (2000, p. 285), according to whom *social care* is to be understood as the following:

> . . .The activities and relations involved in meeting the physical and emotional requirements of dependent adults and children, and the normative,

economic and social frameworks within which these are assigned and carried out.

Looking at care through these dimensions results in an understanding of care, first and foremost, as work that is provided in different dimensions: formal/informal and paid/unpaid. In addition, it allows us to look at how this work is shaped and organized not only through a gendered division of labor but also as a reflection of a shared cultural understanding of what care is supposed to be. Finally, it permits an exploration of the cost of this labor in emotional, organizational, and financial terms. This multidimensional conception of care, in turn, allows for a complex exploration of how the welfare state interacts with, produces, and shapes particular formulations of care organization. Daly and Lewis suggest that an analysis of the welfare state in relation to this dimension should include (1) an investigation of the care infrastructure (provision of care or services); (2) an analysis of the division of labor, responsibility, and costs among the family, the market, the state, and the volunteer/community sector, explicitly looking at the interaction among them; and (3) a study of the way in which welfare state provision disrupts or encourages an existing gendered division of labor (Daly & Lewis, 2000).

Daly and Lewis' formulation is important because it allows us to unearth some of the elements that are at the core of the organization of care that the state can influence through care provision.

This formulation has been further expanded by the literature on comparative *care regimes*, which argues that to fully understand the organization of care and its financing it is crucial to explore how different elements specific to a national context, including the institutional, the regulatory, the political, the social, and the cultural, come together and through these intersections generate different models of care (Bettio & Plantenga, 2004; Da Roit & Weicht, 2013, p. 471; Simonazzi, 2009: 216). This literature, taken together, provides important insights on the many ways in which the state operates as a meso level creating, shaping and organizing the macro level processes generated at the global, regional level described in the section above and the micro level processes of daily interaction between families, im/migrant home eldercare assistants and the elders. Here too as with the previous literature I will not engage with a singular author but highlight how the work of different scholars as a whole (among others Bettio & Plantenga, 2004; Bettio et al., 2006; Daly & Lewis, 2000; Da Roit, 2007; Da Roit & Weicht, 2013; Lyon, 2006; Lyon & Gluckmann, 2008; Shutes & Chiatti, 2012; Simonazzi, 2009; Ungerson & Yeandle, 2007; van Hooren, 2014; Williams & Gavanas, 2008; Williams, 2012) helps to tease out how the state participates in creating and shaping the current organization of home eldercare.

One of the most important elements of analysis that permits an exploration of the way in which the state shapes care provision is the examination of the presence or the absence of social services and the level of difficulty involved in accessing them. When social services for eldercare are absent, families are more likely to look for them in the informal labor market in which, historically, domestic relationships of labor take place. Through this process families are more likely to re-create traditional relationships of domestic labor with which they are familiar instead of seeking new arrangements that may be more specific to eldercare needs.

A second element providing important insights is the structure of support or care infrastructure (services versus cash provision) set in place by the state (Daly & Lewis, 2000; Williams, 2012). States can choose to provide either services or cash provisions; they can provide them universally or only to a select few. In addition, they can choose how to regulate these provisions, for example, in the case of care allowances the state can decide whether to attach rules and regulations or not. Each one of these decisions will have consequences for the way in which care is understood by society at large, and in the way in which care is distributed in terms of labor, costs, and responsibilities between state, family, market, and the voluntary sector. In fact, while the provision of services allows the state more control over the ways in which these services are produced and delivered, cash provisions allow for freer access to the market. Additionally, cash provisions with no rules and regulations attached allow care to be purchased in both the formal and informal labor market, thereby providing opportunity for the expansion of both (Da Roit, 2007; Glucksmann & Lyon, 2006). The choice of instruments can also discourage or encourage existing relationships of care: if, for example, the Italian state suddenly chose to expand care services in regimes of care in which care has always been provided by families, and particularly women in those families, the traditional gendered division of labor could be potentially subverted. Conversely, by providing cash for care the state does not necessarily challenge the cultural and social orientation of care, but by providing ideal notions of "choice" (Ungerson & Yeandle, 2007) may actually exacerbate existing inequalities or create new ones as in the case of the Italian transformation from a "family-centered care model to a "migrant in the family" care model (Bettio et al., 2006).

Furthermore, to fully understand the current organization of care it is critical to understand the distribution of labor, responsibility, and costs spread across the family, the market, the state, and the volunteer/community sector and the consequences that variations in that distribution may entail. Scholars have pointed out how in recent years a process of marketization of care has increasingly changed the distribution of labor, responsibility, and costs among the social actors mentioned above (Shutes & Chiatti, 2012). When this happens the market grows in power, affecting the way in which care is understood. Care, at least in some forms, becomes a product, a commodity to be purchased in the market and in the process it has to become somewhat quantifiable in terms of time and services (Lister et al., 2007; Lyon, 2006). In this process some of the pressure on the family to provide care diminishes, but its costs may increase, creating a new set of problems. Most importantly, however, families are transformed in this process from providers of care into consumers, and, potentially, into employers, and as such they have to learn by themselves how to assess and define the shape, the costs, and the quality of that care. They have to quantify and monetize, and, depending on the size of the cash provision, attempt to extract as much care as possible out of that provision. How families engage in that consumption and in what forms depends greatly on the ways in which the state involves itself in the process. The manner in which the state provides services for this consumption, the ways in which it regulates and shapes the labor market to support it, and how it shapes and regulate labor relations that emerge from it, all affect family engagement in the process.

Finally, as emphasized by Williams (2012), to fully understand how care is organized in a specific national context it is also important to explore how the care regime intersects with the migration and employment regime. The state, in fact, influences the Italian organization of care not only directly but also indirectly. It does so directly by creating policies aimed at attracting im/migrant workers to specific labor markets through a system of quotas and amnesties attached to specific jobs, but it also does so indirectly by, for example, unofficially deskilling workers. Many of my respondents talked about the insurmountable difficulties encountered in trying to have their degrees recognized in Italy. It does so also by tying the provision of the work permit to the presence of a job, which leads workers to take the first job offered to them, independent of working conditions and wages. In addition, by placing the onus of filing amnesties on the employers, the state forces im/migrant workers to shape themselves as "indispensable" to convince families to undertake the difficult and expensive process. As Shutes and Chiatti (2012, p. 399) state:

> *Choice* for migrant workers regarding their entry to and exit from care work is, therefore, conditioned by immigration controls which structure highly unequal relations between migrant care workers and their employers.

Only through a combination of these different approaches and a macrolevel, mesolevel, and microlevel analysis of their interactions is it possible to fully understand how and through what inequalities the current system of home eldercare assistance came into being, how it operates, what are its pros and cons, and in what ways in which it could be transformed in order to provide a more equitable system for the elders, their families, and the workers who care for them.

METHODOLOGY

To study home eldercare assistance I spent 14 months, from August 2003 to September 2004, in Turin, one of the largest cities in Italy, located in the north of the country, where I interviewed 20 academics, trade unionists, nongovernmental organization (NGO) representatives, researchers, and community-based organizers concerned with issues of gender, migration, and work. These interviews, in turn, allowed me to gain access to three different NGOs—Apidad, Benevolentia, and Tierra[8]—that provide a wide variety of services for im/migrant workers, including informal mediation services between families in need of assistance and im/migrant workers looking for work. These organizations helped me contact a large number of both regular and irregular im/migrant women looking for work. In the process I conducted 35 interviews[9] with women of 12 different nationalities, ranging from the Ivory Coast to Albania, from the Philippines to Ecuador, who were working or had worked in the past 6 months as home eldercare assistants and had obtained a work permit. I also had 20 conversations with eldercare workers who were in the country without a work permit, but in order to avoid endangering their migration projects, I did not officially include them in the project. Nevertheless, many of the insights for this book also come from these conversations.

In addition to these interviews, between January 2004 and July 2004 I also did many hours of participant observation at Tierra, assisting the cultural mediator in her weekly meetings with im/migrant women looking for work. Starting in April 2004, I helped conduct a collaborative research project, together with Tierra and ASL4, one of the Turin branches of the national health care system, geared to understanding the needs of Italian families caring for disabled elders. As a result of this project I conducted 26 interviews with family members who were currently taking care of disabled elders either by themselves or with the support of home eldercare assistants. In January 2011 I did 10 follow-up[10] interviews with regional and local public employees, NGOs members, educators, academics, temporary agency managers, and social cooperatives representatives to assess what had changed in the landscape of home eldercare assistance since the economic crisis of 2008 and the period 2009–2014 when unauthorized immigration was officially considered a crime. These conversations and the collection of secondary literature allowed me to gain deeper insights into the changes, or lack thereof, that had occurred in home eldercare assistance since 2004. More detailed information regarding the specifics of the interviews is available in the appendices at the end of the book.

THE ORGANIZATION OF THE BOOK

The chapters in this book are organized in order to reflect the themes outlined earlier in this introduction. Chapter 1 provides an overview of current demographic trends that outlines the progressive "graying" of societies in many areas of the world and it discusses the growing need for long-term care associated with this development. In the process the chapter shows that aging is not an individual issue rather the product of technological, economic and cultural transformations that have taken places over centuries. The chapter then investigates the difficulties that states and families encounter in providing such care due in part to changes at the political, the social and the cultural level such as increased female participation in the labor market, increased geographical mobility, progressive deconstruction of extended and even nuclear families and a restructuring of welfare states linked to current neoliberal ideologies. Finally, the chapter analyzes the impact of adopting market-oriented ideologies and mechanisms to address the growing need for long-term care and its different outcomes in different societies of the Global North. Chapter 2 opens with a description of the growing role of female im/migrant labor in the provision of home eldercare assistance and then proceeds to explore how this labor force became available. In particular, the chapter explores how different actors—such as sending and receiving countries, supranational organizations such as the IMF and the World Bank, and regional ones such as the European Union—participate in generating, managing, and sustaining migration flows from the Global South to the Global North. Through this analysis the chapter describes global trends that have contributed to what some scholars have defined as the new division of reproductive labor, the growth of what are known as Global Care Chains, and the "feminization" of migration processes.

Chapter 3 continues the exploration of home eldercare work by locating it in the specifics of the Italian case. This chapter explores how global and regional macroprocesses become embedded in the local reality of one specific country, in this case Italy, generating new realities, new jobs, and new economic and social relations. Specifically, the chapter looks at how the feminization of migration generated through political and economic transformations both in sending and receiving countries came to intersect with the growing need for short-term and long-term eldercare in Italy, a need generated not only by demographic processes but also by cultural, social, and economic transformations. In addition, the chapter explores the role that migration policies, both at the regional and national level, play in creating a segmented, gendered, and racialized labor force.

Chapter 4 investigates the reasons behind Italian families' decision to become employers of home eldercare assistants. It does so first by exploring the current organization of long-term eldercare in Italy: who provides it, in what terms, the impact of care provision on caregivers' lives and the lives of their families, together with its costs at both the economic and emotional level for all the actors involved. It continues by analyzing the support that the state provides to families both in terms of services and cash provisions and how this support increasingly pushes families to seek care support in the informal labor market. Finally, it concludes by looking at how family caregivers are actively transformed into employers.

Chapter 5 outlines how im/migrant women from different racial and ethnic, class, professional and educational backgrounds are transformed into *home eldercare assistants*. The chapter shows how this transformation happens through daily discourse and practices at different levels: global and local, private, and public. It also shows how discourse and practices help to create a hierarchy in the labor market along racial/ethnic, national, and cultural lines.

Chapter 6 describes the routines of both live-in and live-out workers throughout a typical day on the job. In the process the chapter reveals that home eldercare assistance while often being portrayed simply as an offshoot of domestic labor is in reality a different occupation with its own set of skills, goals, and priorities. In addition, it shows that while this job is often depicted as unskilled in reality it requires that the workers take on, during their long work day, different roles, each requiring a different set of skills: from maid to chaperone, from nurse to therapist, and from cook to spiritual counselor. Finally the chapter includes a discussion of the different dimensions of eldercare according to the women who provide it.

Chapter 7 delves into the emotional labor required in this occupation and how the relationships that develop on the job affect the relationship of power between the workers and the elders. Although it is true that emotional labor allows families to extract more work from the immigrant workers, at times the emotional attachment may work in favor of the workers and guarantee them a stronger bargaining power in terms of wages, work hours, and help in obtaining a residency permit. In addition, a discussion of emotional labor and the ways in which it is enacted through daily routines permits a deeper understanding of how gender roles are both transformed and renegotiated in home eldercare assistance.

Finally, the concluding chapter brings together some of the themes analyzed throughout the book, provides a discussion of the findings, and includes a discussion of what a more equitable redistribution of care could look like.

NOTES

1 *Nonna* in Italian means *grandma*, a term usually used only by family members. However, im/migrant home eldercare assistants use it often to define the elderly person for whom they work. A further discussion of this term will be undertaken in Chapter 7.

2 I use the term im/migrant instead of choosing to settle on either immigrant or migrant to indicate that in Italy there are both immigrants and migrants. Some people come with the intention to settle, if not permanently, then long-term, whereas others participate in circulatory migration.

3 The term "badante" is a term that was used for the first time in the Bossi-Fini immigration law to define im/migrant workers, mostly women, less often men, who provide eldercare services for Italian families. The term has been contested because in the past the verb "badare" (to take care of)

was used in reference to animals and therefore many consider it offensive for both the care providers and the care receivers. Feminists, in particular, have been pushing for the adoption of the term "care assistants." For this reason from now on I use the term "home eldercare assistants" instead of "badanti."

4 Although women are the majority in this occupation, there is also a smaller male presence. More specific data on this presence are presented in Chapter 3.

5 To compare it with the previous model of care that was a "familial" one.

6 A recent study suggests that in Italy "the migrant share of the overall care workforce exceeds 40 percent and is 4–5 times higher than its share in the rest of the labor market" (Cangiano, 2014, p. 138).

7 This section is not a literature review, but simply an exploration of the ways in which the literature has helped to shape this project. Both literatures are explored more extensively in Chapters 2 and 3.

8 To protect the privacy of the interviewees I used pseudonyms instead of the real names of these organizations. Apidad and Benevolentia are two Catholic organizations, whereas Tierra is a feminist organization composed of Italian and immigrant women.

9 To respect the privacy and the confidentiality of all the people involved in this project the real names of the interviewees have been changed to fictional ones.

10 In this case too all the names have been changed to pseudonyms to protect the privacy of the interviewees.

Caring for a Living

1

THE CHANGING LANDSCAPE OF ELDERCARE

As discussed in the introduction, the *graying* of the population is a global phenomenon. In fact, according to the United Nations Population Division (UNPD), the overall number of the population aged 60 years and over is projected to increase from 810 million today to over two billion in 2050. [United Nations Population Division (UNPD), 2012a]. The degree of this growth is somewhat staggering; United Nations Population Fund (UNFPA) data show that in the past 10 years alone "the number of people aged 60 or over has risen by 178 million--equivalent to nearly the entire population of Pakistan, the sixth most populous country in the world" (UNFPA, 2012, p. 20). This growth in the elderly population is accompanied by another important phenomenon: the aging of the old population itself. The UNPD data show that the oldest old population (80 years or over) is the fastest growing age segment of the older population and it is expected to grow from the current figure of 69 million to 400 million in 2050 (Harper & Leeson, 2009; UNPD, 2012a). Although this segment now accounts for 14% of the population, it is projected to reach 20% by 2050. Currently 40% of the people over 80 years old live in Asia, with some 16% in China alone; 30% live in Europe, and 13% live in the United States. In addition, the number of centenarians (men and women aged 100 years or over) is growing even faster, and is projected to increase 10-fold, from approximately 343,000 in 2012 to 3.2 million by 2050 (Timonen, 2008; UNPD, 2012a). This tilting of the population toward an older range is not necessarily a negative development, but it is certainly one that needs acknowledgment and preparedness, because it creates a whole new set of issues with respect to care. To better understand aging and its many dimensions in this chapter I will provide some background to this phenomenon exploring the demographic, economic, political, and cultural processes behind its development. In addition, I will also explore some of the new needs that aging, in combination with an extended life span, is generating.

AGING AS A GLOBAL PHENOMENON

The shift toward an older population, although global, is not happening at the same rate everywhere in the world. As of today the greatest concentration of the population 60 years and older continues to be found in the wealthier regions of the world: one in five persons in Europe; one in nine persons in Asia, Latin America, and the Caribbean; and one in 16 persons in Africa, but these proportions are expected to change substantially by 2050 [United Nations Department of Economic and Social Affairs (UNDESA), 2013; World Health Organization (WHO), 2012a]. Today, almost two in three people aged 60 years and over reside in the global North, with the highest concentrations in Japan, Italy, and Germany followed by the countries of Northern Europe. By 2050 four in five people aged 60 years and over will live in the global South, and the list of countries with the highest concentration will change significantly, including countries such as Cuba and South Korea (UNDESA, 2013), and countries such as Chile, China, and Iran will contain a greater proportion of older people than the United States (UNFPA, 2012; WHO, 2012a). In other words, although the countries of the global North currently have the oldest population profiles, the largest numbers of older people—and the fastest aging populations—are actually in the global South [National Institute for Aging and the National Institutes of Health (NIA-NIH), 2010). Table 1.1 provides an overview of the aging process at the regional level, whereas Table 1.2 provides a list of countries in which the largest share of the population is currently aged 60 years and over as well as a projection for 2050.

Table 1.1. Average Annual Growth Rate of the Population Aged 60 Years and Older (%)

Region of the World	Population Aged 60 and Older					
	Number (Thousands)		Proportion of Total Population (Percentage)		Share of Persons 80 Years and Older (Percentage of Aged Population)	
	2012	2050	2012	2050	2012	2050
Africa	59,782	215,249	6	10	8	10
Asia	446,974	1,252,588	11	24	12	19
Europe	166,397	241,828	22	34	20	28
Latin America and the Caribbean	63,064	187,869	10	25	15	22
Northern America	67,597	120,797	19	27	20	30
Oceania	5,928	13,006	16	24	18	27

Source: National Institute for Aging and the National Institutes of Health (2010).

Table 1.2. Countries with the Highest Shares of Population 60 Years and over in 2011 and 2050 (Percent) (Among Countries with a 2011 Population of 1 Million or More)

2011		2050	
Japan	31	Japan	42
Italy	27	Portugal	40
Germany	26	Bosnia and Herzegovina	40
Finland	25	Cuba	39
Sweden	25	Republic of Korea	39
Bulgaria	25	Italy	38
Greece	25	Spain	38
Portugal	24	Singapore	38
Belgium	24	Germany	38
Croatia	24	Switzerland	37

Source: Global Population Aging: Peril or Promise World Economic Forum (2012) from data provided by the United Nations Population Division (2011).

Even among wealthier countries, the speed of the process varies greatly due to different social, cultural, and political conditions. Classical demographers argue that the aging of the population is the result of a long-term process called the *demographic transition,* which summarizes historical patterns initially observed in Europe but is somewhat useful in explaining shifts in population in other countries as well (Lee, 2003; Lee, 2011, p. 569).

During this transition, populations move from high and fluctuating levels of fertility and mortality to low and relatively stable levels of both (Lee, 2003, p. 170; Timonen, 2008). Typically the shift happens in three consecutive phases. In the first phase, mortality begins to decline, whereas fertility remains high. In this stage mortality tends to decline most at the youngest ages, creating an increase in the proportions of children and raising the overall child dependency ratios. In the second phase, fertility begins to decline, lowering the child dependency ratio, and the working-age population grows faster than the population as a whole. In this phase the total dependency ratio, the ratio between those of working age and those of nonworking age, tends to decline as well. In the third phase, societies experience an increase in longevity that generally leads to a rapid increase in the elderly population, and lower fertility rates slow the growth of the working age population. In this phase the old-age dependency ratio rises rapidly, as does the total dependency ratio (Lee, 2003, p. 182).

Although explanatory, this three-phase model tends to be an ideal type because the transition between lower mortality and declining fertility does not always happen in the same way or for the same reasons. In France and the United States, for example, fertility began to decline first (Lee, 2003), whereas in lower-income countries the temporal gap between the decline in mortality and fertility has been very small and the two processes may overlap (Timonen,

2008). Although classical demographic transition theory suggests that mortality and fertility decline in an almost fixed pattern, in reality there is a great deal of variation. Notwithstanding these criticisms, this model provides useful inferences about how mortality and fertility impact various populations, and offers some insights into what the future may hold.

A BRIEF TIMELINE OF THE DEMOGRAPHIC TRANSITION

At the moment the demographic transition is an open-ended process, but it is possible to provide a basic timeline for its development. The global demographic transition started in northwest Europe during the nineteenth century when mortality began to decline. This decline led to a rapid rise in population growth, a growth that reached its apex in the twentieth century. During this time, lower children's mortality led to an increase in the younger population, which in turn led to a rise in the child dependency ratio. This trend intensified as these children entered their reproductive years, while their parents' high fertility rate remained unchanged (Boongarts, 2009; Lee, 2003). The next phase of the demographic transition started toward the end of the nineteenth century and lasted until the middle of the twentieth century. In this phase, Europe (Eastern and Western) and a few other countries including the United States, Canada, Australia, New Zealand, Argentina, and Uruguay began to experience a drop in fertility rates as well as a decline in mortality. This drop continued until the 1930s–1940s at which point the fertility rate of Europe fell to replacement levels of 2.1, whereas mortality continued to decline. Fertility continued to decline in Europe, with the exception of a short-lived baby boom in the mid-1960s, reaching levels of 1.5 or below during the 1980s in what has been termed the second demographic transition (Harper, 2005; Van de Kaa, 1987).

Outside Western countries the demographic transition followed a different pattern. In most of the world the decline in mortality did not start until the early twentieth century, but then accelerated dramatically after World War II. The result was a jump in population growth that peaked in most societies in the late 1950s and 1960s and, at times, exceeded 2.5% or 3% per year (Reher, 2012, p. 11). These countries experienced the fastest improvements in childhood health, while also making impressive gains in life expectancy. In non-Western countries, however, the decline in mortality was not followed closely by a decline in fertility. On the contrary, total fertility rates increased and the result was a jump in population growth that peaked in most societies in the late 1950s–1960s (Reher, 2012, p. 12). In these countries the decline in fertility started in the mid-1960s or later. However, since World War II low-income countries have typically made more rapid transitions to lower fertility than high-income countries; the total fertility rate over the period 1960–1999 plummeted from 6 to 2.7 in Latin America and from 6.14 to 3.14 in Asia. In Africa the total fertility rate declined moderately from 6.55 in 1960 to 5.0 in 1999 (Lee, 2003). In India the total fertility rate declined from 6.0 in 1966 to 3.6 in 1992 and then it dropped even further, with the total fertility rate having reached 2.6 births per woman by 2008 (James, 2011).

MORTALITY DECLINES

The world's demographic transition began around the 1800s in Northwest Europe when mortality began a secular decline. This trend then expanded over time to other parts of the world, becoming significant in many low-income countries only at the beginning of the twentieth century. The first phase of the decline in mortality was connected to reductions in contagious and infectious diseases usually spread through air and water. However, although the decline in the number of deaths started with the development of vaccine and preventive medicine, it was also linked to better nutrition, increased public health measures, and improved personal hygiene. Increases in income had positive effects on the overall health of the population (Lee, 2003, p. 171, Riley, 2005), and the decline in mortality in this first phase was mostly due to a reduction in children's mortality (Timonen, 2008). More recent gains in life expectancy have been made at the other end of the age spectrum as a result of a progressive decrease in chronic and degenerative diseases, namely heart disease and cancer, thereby reducing mortality at older ages (Riley, 2001). This decrease is mostly linked to changes in lifestyle and behavior, including reductions in smoking, alcohol use, and the consumption of animal fats (Harper, 2005). In the past few decades, biomedical research has played an increasingly important part in extending the life expectancy of the world's population, and it continues to be an important factor in analysis of mortality rates (Lee, 2003, p. 170).

The declines in mortality described above did not start in lower-income countries until sometime in the twentieth century, but once started the gains in life expectancy were, in some areas, quite rapid. According to Ronald Lee, for example, life expectancy in India rose from around 24 years in 1920 to 62 years in 2003. In China, life expectancy rose from 41 years in 1950–1955 to 70 years in 1995–1999 (Lee, 2003, p. 170).

FERTILITY DECLINES

Fertility began to decline dramatically in several European countries in the 1870s and this process continued steadily until the 1920s (Lee, 2003). During this 50-year span, birth rates declined by 44% in England, 37% in Germany, 32% in Sweden and Finland, and 26% in France, and by the 1930s and 1940s most of Europe had fallen to replacement levels (Harper & Leeson, 2009; Galor,

2004). However, the decline in fertility came to a temporary halt after World War II when there were a number of baby booms and busts in different areas of the world (Bloom, Boersch-Supan, McGee, & Atsushi, 2011; Lee, 2003). After that period of growth, fertility began to weaken again, causing what some have defined as the "second fertility transition," in which fertility dropped below replacement levels in many industrial nations reaching an average of 1.5 children per woman (Van de Kaa, 1987). Over time, this trend extended to all areas of Europe and also to other high-income countries such as Canada, Australia, and Japan (Harper 2009). The United States has a total fertility rate of 1.9, which though slightly higher, is not high enough to reach replacement level (World Bank, 2014).

The countries of the global South, on the other hand, started their transitions to lower levels of fertility in the mid-1960s or later, but once they started transitions they progressed much faster than countries of the global North (Lee, 2003). The pace of these declines has surprised even demographers, who were not expecting a process that took over a century in countries such as France to occur in a matter of 20 to 30 years in countries such as South Korea (NIA-NIH, 2007). Declines in fertility rates have been most rapid in Asia, North Africa, and Latin America, but as in the case of mortality, the process was not uniform. Between the early 1960s and the late 1990s the largest fertility declines occurred in Asia (–52%) and Latin America (–55%), with the smallest in sub-Saharan Africa (–15%) (Boongarts, 2001). Differences among countries are even larger, with some completing the transition to replacement fertility in record time (e.g., China, Hong Kong, Singapore, South Korea), whereas others (mostly in sub-Saharan Africa) have seen little change in reproductive behavior (Boongarts, 2002). According to the UNPD, today 42% of the world's population resides in low-fertility countries, another 40% lives in intermediate-fertility countries, and only 18% is located in high-fertility countries (Figure 1.1). Geographically high-fertility countries are concentrated in Africa (39 out of 55 have high fertility), with nine in Asia, six in Oceania, and four in Latin America. Low-fertility countries include all of Europe except Iceland and Ireland, 19 countries out of 51 in Asia, 14 out of 39 in the Americas, two in Africa (Mauritius and Tunisia), and one in Oceania (Australia) (UNPD, 2011, pp. 1–2).

The causes of the decline in fertility are unclear, but different theories provide different explanations. Standard demographic transition theory, for example, suggests that the decline in fertility happens in response to the decline in mortality. Once parents realize that their offspring are more likely to survive, they choose to give birth to a smaller number of children. Some social scientists instead argue that the decline in fertility rates is connected to increasing technical innovations in contraception together with transmission of information and ideas regarding fertility control. Other scholars, mainly historians and sociologists, have attempted to explain the decline through attitudinal changes often linked to modernization and westernization that resulted in smaller, nuclear

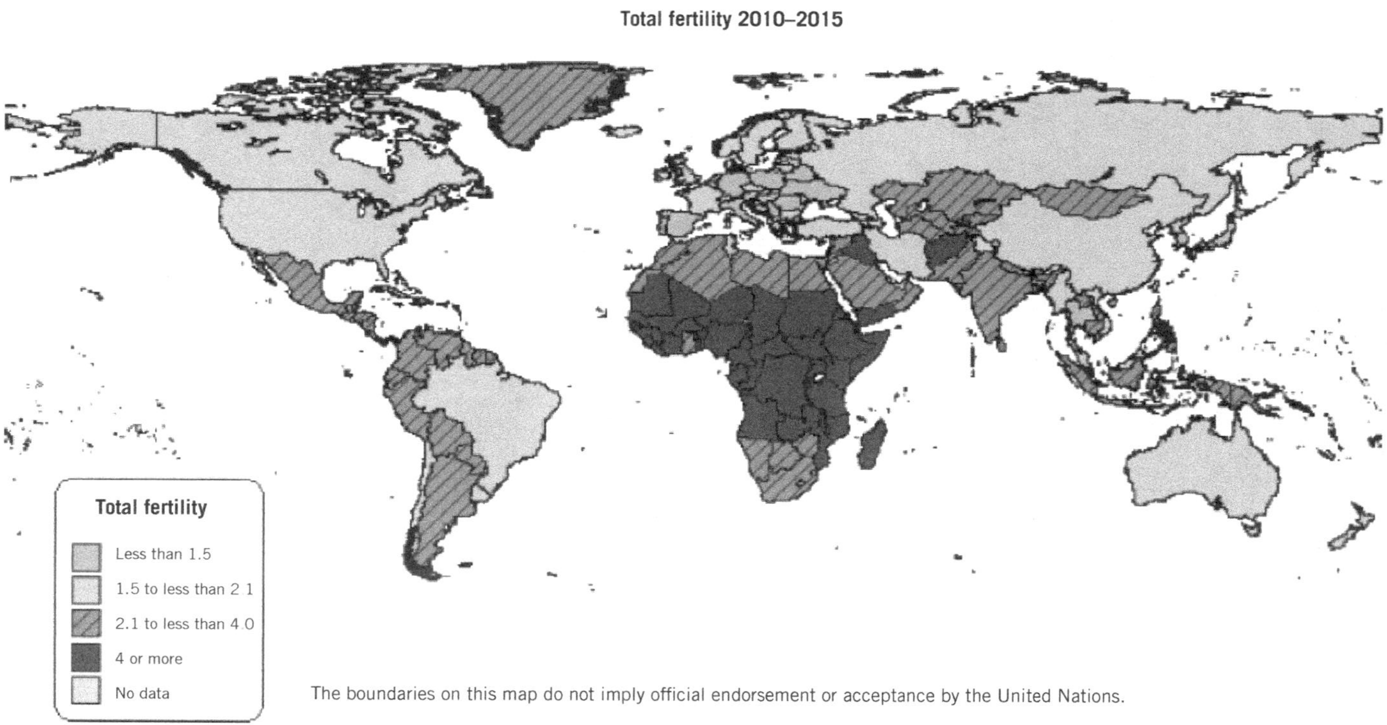

Figure 1.1. Countries and areas classified by fertility level. *Source*: United Nations Department of Economic and Social Affairs, Population Division (2013b) *Fertility Levels and Trends As Assessed in the 2012 Revision of World Population Prospects.*

families. Feminist theorists in particular have attempted to explain this phenomenon by looking at the complex relationship between sexuality, personal lives, and social policy (Folbre, 1983). Economists, on the other hand, have focused on the increasing cost of having children as a possible explanation for the decline in fertility, particularly after the passage from an agricultural to an industrial society. Harper (2009, p. 436) states that "Capital-investment theory suggests that the need to invest in education as skill-based labor markets arose during the industrial revolution resulted in parents lowering fertility to invest more in fewer high quality children." Others explained the decline by linking it to the increasing difficulties that women in contemporary industrialized societies face in combining childrearing with education and career, whereas cultural theories suggested that lower fertility is the outcome of a radical change in fundamental norms and values with regard to the need and desire to have children. According to these theories, increased individualism and consumerism together with a strong emphasis on quality of life and leisure, a desire for self-actualization and freedom, together with a retreat from commitment may reduce the number of births in a given society (Boongarts, 2002; Harper, 2009; McDonald, 2000).

Although all of these theories offer potentially valuable explanations for the decline in fertility across the world, there seems to be no agreement on which potential explanatory factors weigh more heavily than others. Not to mention that in some cases declines in fertility were neither an automatic response nor a choice, but were imposed from above as in the case of the forced sterilizations of the 1960s and 1970s, the Chinese "one child policy," or development agencies strongly supporting population control operating in many countries of the Global South. In other words, it is fair to say that the answer to the decline in fertility varies from society to society, depending on the geopolitical, economic, and cultural condition of each country.

LIFE EXPECTANCY AND HEALTHY LIFE EXPECTANCY

The data we just looked at provide us with a sense of the transformations that have affected our societies over time. A particularly important element of these changes is increased life expectancy, which grows when morbidity and mortality are postponed to older ages. In most parts of the world people are living significantly longer lives than in previous decades; data from the United Nations Population Division show that although average life expectancy at birth was just 48 years between 1950 and 1955, in 1995–2000 it had grown to 65 years and it is currently estimated to reach 78 years by 2050 (Bloom et al., 2011; UNPD, 2013). However, once again, the process is not even. The first difference is at the gender level; women tend to live longer than men. According to the UNFPA (2012, p. 27) "In 2012, for every 100 women aged 60, there were 84 men.

The proportion of women rises further with age. For every 100 women aged 80 or over worldwide, there are only 61 men."

The gap between the two groups is high enough that scholars and policy makers have begun to talk about *the feminization of aging* (Davidson, DiGiacomo, & McGrath, 2011). And, of course, there are large discrepancies between different areas of the world. According to the World Health Organization, "In 2009 life expectancy at birth globally was 68 years ranging from 57 years in low income countries to 80 years in high income countries giving a ratio of 1.4 between the two income groups" (WHO, 2012a). The inequity in life expectancy becomes even clearer when looking at the different regions. Africa and parts of Oceania were the two areas of the world with the lowest life expectancies at birth in 1950–1955, and the same remains true today. Whereas average life expectancy has increased in Melanesia, Micronesia, and Polynesia to 64 years in 2005–2010, in Africa it remains only 55 years. Asia, Latin America, and the Caribbean, on the other hand, have made rapid gains in life expectancy over the past 60 years, reaching an average of 70 years, but they have not yet reached the levels of the wealthy regions of the world (Europe, the United States, Canada, Australia, and Japan) where life expectancy has reached an average of 80 years and over (UNPD, 2012b). Variation is not limited to geographic areas. Great differences, in fact, can be found at the national level. Table 1.3 lists the 30 countries with the highest life expectancies in 2012.

As we can see from Table 1.3, the majority of the countries in this list belong to the global North, suggesting that although aging is a global process, high life expectancy is still closely associated with high levels of income.[1] This observation is further supported by the Department of Economic and Social Affairs of

Table 1.3. Life Expectancy for Males and Females

Country	M	F	Country	M	F	Country	M	F
1. Monaco	85.74	93.77	11. Liechtenstein	79.37	84.19	21. Netherlands	78.84	83.08
2. Macau	81.47	87.54	12. Canada	78.89	84.21	22. Bermuda	77.6	84.1
3. Japan	80.57	87.43	13. Jersey	79.05	84.04	23. Cayman Islands	78.12	83.51
4. Singapore	81.47	86.2	14. France	78.35	84.73	24. Isle of Man	79.17	82.47
5. San Marino	80.55	85.81	15. Spain	78.26	84.47	25. New Zealand	78.7	82.81
6. Andorra	80.4	84.74	16. Sweden	78.86	83.63	26. Ireland	78.07	82.69
7. Guernsey	79.57	85.04	17. Switzerland	78.34	84.16	27. Norway	77.65	83.14
8. Hong Kong	79.39	85.05	18. Israel	78.88	83.36	28. Germany	77.93	82.58
9. Australia	79.48	84.45	19. Iceland	78.81	83.29	29. Jordan	78.82	81.61
10. Italy	79.24	84.63	20. Anguilla	78.42	83.63	30. United Kingdom	78.05	82.4

Source: Data elaborated from the CIA World Factbook (2012).

the United Nations Population Division (2010a:1): "In high- and upper-middle-income countries, 78 per cent of deaths occur at age 60 or over and 40 per cent at age 80 and over. In lower-middle class countries, the equivalent proportions are 66 per cent and 24 per cent."

However, while future trends in life expectancy cannot be certain due to the many variables that can potentially affect them, projections suggest that life span will continue to increase worldwide, reaching an all time high of 81.1 years in 2095-2100 (UN DESA PD 2010b).

While increases in life expectancy are certainly one of the greatest achievements of the twenty-first century, these achievement do not necessarily imply an independent and healthy life or guarantee a greater quality of life. Recent studies investigating this issue report discrepancies between life expectancy and healthy life expectancies. To clarify, the first term refers to the average number of years that a newborn is expected to live if current mortality rates continue to apply, whereas the second term refers to the average number of years that a person can expect to live in "full health" by taking into account years lived in less than full health due to disease and/or injury (WHO, 2010, pp. 3–4). Although looking at increased life expectancy may fill us with wonder regarding our ability to extend human life, this second indicator may reduce the feeling. A recent study[2] conducted by the Institute for Health Metrics and Evaluation and other academic partners states (Salomon et al., 2012, pp. 2144–2147):

> In 2010, global male HALE (Healthy Life Expectancy) at birth was 59 years and global female HALE at birth was 63.2 years. Across countries in 2010, male HALE at birth ranged from 27.8 years in Haiti to 70.6 years in Japan. Female HALE at birth ranged from 37.1 years in Haiti to 75.5 years in Japan. . . [Overall] the difference between life expectancy and healthy life expectancy was 8.5 years for the male population, and 10 years for the female population.

This study reveals a fairly long gap between the time at which men and women can consider themselves in good health and the time of their death. According to the same study, this gap tends to increase in countries with higher life expectancy. The data, in fact, show that as life expectancy increases, so does the gap between life expectancy and healthy life expectancy (2149). In Italy, for example, a country with a relatively high life expectancy (78.9 for males and 83.9 for females), the gap between life expectancy and HALE in 2010 was as high as 10 years for males and almost 12 years for females (68.3 and 71.9 years, respectively). A similar pattern is evident in the case of the United States, where life expectancy in 2010 was 75.9 years for males and 80.5 years for females, with a HALE of 66.2 and 69.5 years, respectively. In Zambia, on the other hand, where life expectancy is 54.3 years for males and 57.3 years for females, the gap between the two is smaller, with a HALE of 46.8 years for males and 48.7 years for women. The Global Burden of Disease (GBD) study suggests that these discrepancies are due to the changing causes of death across the world. According to the GBD study, population aging, and to a lesser extent population growth, in general, have contributed to an increase in deaths from non-communicable diseases (e.g., among others: ischemic heart disease, cancer, diabetes, depression). This increase in turn has raised the numbers of healthy years that men and women lose due to these conditions. This is particularly true for Australia, Japan, the United States, and the wealthy countries of Europe where non-communicable diseases are particularly prominent (IHME, 2013).

In addition, the comparison between life expectancy and HALE also highlights an important new element: while women live longer than men, overall they seem to lose more years than men to sickness and morbidity. This difference may expose women, who in general have lower incomes than men, to a higher level of dependency in their older ages, potentially creating both health and economic impacts.

The data we just examined highlight two important points: on the one hand they emphasize that longer living is not necessarily a synonym for healthy living. Even though we are certainly making progress in increasing the life span across the globe, the data on healthy life expectancy show that there will be times during that increased life span when people will not be able to live independently or will require some kind of support. In addition, they show that periods of disability requiring support may range from a very short time to extended periods of time lasting as long as 10 years and more. On the other hand, the data highlight that although aging is certainly a growing global trend, high life expectancy is still closely associated with high levels of income. By this point in the analysis it is fair to state that while aging and issues associated with it will become dramatically relevant in countries of the global South in the next 20 to 40 years, it is the global North that is currently grappling with issues of aging. Given this, from here on I will focus more specifically on these countries, without forgetting, however, that other countries are already approaching similar trajectories.

THE INCREASED NEED FOR ELDERCARE

Together with aging, one of the fastest growing issues of the twenty-first century is the increased need for long-term care for the elderly. As seen in the previous section, there is a positive relationship between increased life expectancy and years lost to disability. Periods of disability together with a general decline in physical and/or cognitive functioning related to the general process of aging do increase the level of dependency that aging men and women will experience in their lifetime, particularly in the older age groups. In this landscape, short-term and long-term care services for elders, whether provided in institutions or by family and community, have become essential to the well-being of many (Figure 1.2).

As we will see in detail in Chapter 4, the care services needed by the elderly population have many dimensions that may vary over time, but in the health and policy literature they are described as activities of daily living (ADLs) and instrumental activities of daily living (IADLs). ADLs refer to a range of services aimed at helping the elders accomplish basic personal functions such as bathing, dressing, eating, toileting, and getting in and out of beds and chairs. IADLs are often offered in conjunction with ADLs and are intended to provide support with household chores and the management of everyday life, such as grocery shopping, paying bills, medication management, and transportation (Stone, 2011, p. 3; Timonen, 2008). Care for the elders may also range from companionship and emotional support to extensive 24/7 supervision for those affected by dementia or Alzheimer's disease. In addition to these long-term care services, elders may also need short-term support during a hospital stay or upon discharge after an operation or a serious illness (Da Roit, 2006; Timonen, 2008).

Societies of the global North, however, are ill prepared to deal with this increased need and are currently struggling to provide answers to some of the following questions: Who will provide this new and increased range of care services? Under what terms and conditions would they do so? Who is responsible for paying for these services? The anxiety created by these uncertainties is affecting an increasingly large number of states around the world to the point that it has generated a language of crisis, causing some to declare

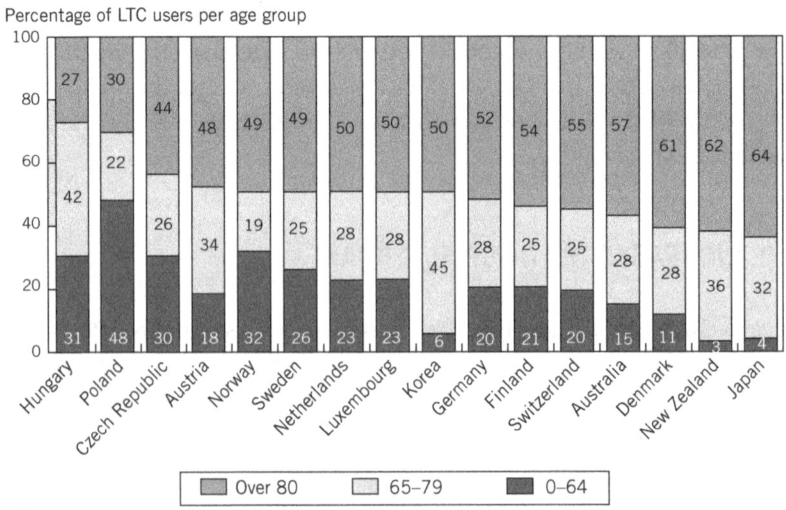

Figure 1.2. Share of long-term care users by age, 2008. *Source*: OECD (Colombo et al. 2011, p. 41).

that we are experiencing, or will experience in the near future, an *eldercare crisis*. The anxiety concerning the provision of eldercare is further reinforced by the fact that previous forms of care provision are no longer tenable. To this day, most long-term care for elders across the world has been shouldered by families, and more specifically by the women in these families (Silverstein & Giarrusso, 2010), but recent social, economic, cultural, and political developments are affecting these traditional arrangements. One of these factors is the increased participation of women[3] in the labor market. In the United States female participation increased from 34% in 1950 to 60% in the late 90s, almost doubling over the course of 50 years. Although the rate has had a slight decline to a 2014 level of 57% the increase largely remains (Goldin, 1989; BLS, 2015b). Europe experienced a similar growth, albeit with a great deal of variation among countries[4] (Lutz, 2006; Standing, 1999). Overall, however, the rate of employment for women went from an average of 39% in 1970s to 52% in 1998 reaching 63.5% in 2014. (European Commission 2015, Van Hooren, 2011:3). Similar patterns are also present in other countries of the global North: female labor participation grew in Japan from 52.7% in 1981 to 66.0% in 2014, in Australia from 52.2% to 70.5%, and in Canada from 59.2% to 74.2% (OECD, 2015). In all cases once women entered the labor market the unpaid work that they once performed invisibly in the home had to be redistributed. However, as women entered the realm of paid labor outside the home, men's behavior remained relatively unchanged (Mattingly & Bianchi, 2003; Craig, 2006). Some men may take on more of the child care and housework (Deutsch, 1999; Hochschild, 2003), but most of the responsibility for social reproduction still falls upon women.

Many scholars (Crittenden, 2001; Folbre, 2001; Hochschild, 1997; among others) have pointed out that notwithstanding women's increased participation in the labor market, the workplace is still centered on the *ideal-worker* norm, which assumes that workers dedicate their lives to work, unencumbered by family responsibilities. As a consequence, women often put motherhood on hold, postponing childbearing until later in life. This deferred motherhood often results in women being caught in a lifelong time bind; as soon as they finish raising their children, they find themselves under pressure to care for elderly relatives. For some, the claims on their time overlap (Daly & Standing, 2001), creating even more strain in the already tenuous balance between work and family time.

The changing position of women in the labor market, although critical in generating a higher demand for paid care service, is by no means the only reason behind this so-called eldercare crisis. Other cultural, demographic, political, and social changes affect the way care is provided as well. In many countries, notions of family and household dynamics have been changing. More and more societies around the world have experienced the downfall of extended family systems and the resulting nuclearization of households on the one hand and the increase of new atypical household forms on the other (Daly & Standing, 2001). In addition, these societies have seen an increase in the number of single heads of household. Formerly stable structures such as families and kin networks have therefore become more precarious, adding an element of instability to the traditional organization of care. In current circumstances, old norms of behavior, expectations, and reciprocity are no longer easily fulfilled, creating a growing sense of insecurity. This problem is intensified by the fact that contemporary societies tend to be more mobile. The age of globalization has pushed and/or allowed for greater mobility, so that individuals and households are increasingly cut off from extended families, neighbors, and traditional communities. This mobility makes it harder for people to access informal networks of care or, perhaps more importantly, to care for distant family members (Daly & Standing, 2001; Saraceno, 2003a; Timonen, 2008).

Demographic changes can also affect eldercare provision. As noted in the previous section, countries of the global North have experienced an overall decline in fertility with the exception of the baby booms of the 1960s. This decline has multiple consequences. On one hand there is a growing number of elderly people who are childless, and therefore likely to require support from outside the family, and on the other there are fewer daughters, daughters-in-law, and female relatives to provide care. Given that for the most part eldercare continues to be shouldered by women, the deficit in the numbers of potential female caregivers is a matter of serious concern.

The result of all these concomitant developments is that an increased demand for eldercare has corresponded with a decline in the ability of the family to provide it. This decline has had particularly grave consequences in countries in which the welfare state has always relied on families to provide care, such as Italy, Spain, Greece, and Japan, but it also affects other societies around the world.

WELFARE STATE RESTRUCTURING AND THE MARKETIZATION OF CARE

In addition to cultural, social, and demographic developments, care provision and its organization have also been affected by the restructuring of welfare states. Starting in the last quarter of the twentieth century, pressures to reduce and control social spending and an increasing enthusiasm for neoliberal ideas have led policy makers to seek cost-effective and cheaper means of delivering services, which resulted in decentralization, changes in welfare provisions, and a focus on strategies involving privatization and marketization of services (Bergqvist & Nyberg, 2002; Daly, 2001; Knijn, 2001; Pavolini & Ranci, 2008; Yeandle & Ungerson, 2007). The growing interest in market and market-based services generated by neoliberalism was also supported by two parallel trends: a growing desire on the part of disabled and elderly people (at least in the United States) to obtain more independence and control over the conditions of their own dependency (Glendinning, 2008; Rabiee, 2013) and a progressive acknowledgment by policy makers and civil society at large that care and its provision could no longer be considered simply a *women's private issue* but that instead it is a matter that needs to be addressed as a *workers' issue* (Williams, 2012).

In response to these different but converging developments welfare states began to explore ways to reshape their role and their relationship to long-term care. Traditionally, among welfare states of the Global North, people in need of care were provided with invalidity pensions and/or health and rehabilitation services. However, these programs were not designed for large numbers of people or for long-term needs, not to mention that they were considered too costly by many states (Pavolini & Ranci, 2008). In addition, during the same period of time there was growing support among policy makers, health practitioners, and social workers for encouraging elderly people to remain in their homes instead of entering institutions (OECD, 2011). Labeled *"Ageing in Place"* (OECD, 2005), this goal has been advocated by many governments both on economic and humanitarian grounds; caring for the elders at home helps reduce expensive institutional care and, at the same time, it is alleged to improve the quality of life for elders (Aronson & Neysmith, 1996, p. 60). Aging in place is believed to improve the daily lives of the elders by promoting independence and autonomy, strengthening feelings of attachment and connections to social support, such as friends and family, as well as fostering a sense of familiarity and security (Wiles, Leibing, Guberman, Reeve, & Allen, 2011). Although the merits of the humanitarian argument are still under investigation (see San Antonio, Eckert, & Simon-Rusinowitz, 2006), the economic argument has been at the center of many Western social policies. Since the early 1970s there has been an increasing tendency in the United States, Canada, and Western Europe to transfer caregiving out of hospitals and institutions to cheaper providers, namely unpaid family members or paid homecare workers. This process, which Glazer (1993) defined as *work transfer*,[5] contributed to governmental attempts to cut public spending. Healthcare policies are organized to ensure that fewer people with chronic health problems are cared for in institutions, that people with acute or terminal medical conditions are discharged as quickly as possible from expensive hospital care, and that elderly citizens and their families choose homes over institutions (Aronson & Neysmith, 1996; Palese, Oliverio, Girardo, Fabbro, & Saiani, 2004).

To support this new ideology many countries of the Global North began to shy away from traditional forms of support (or as in the case of familialist welfare states from relying exclusively on family care) and instead began to offer individuals cash payments to purchase care services. Countries such as the United Kingdom, the Netherlands, Germany, Italy, Austria, Israel, and Japan have adopted different forms of care allowances, direct payments, and social insurance to allow elderly and disabled people to buy support and assistance (OECD, 2011; Williams, 2012, 365). Austria, for example, adopted the Federal Care Allowance Act in 1993 while France introduced cash allowances in 1997 (Martin & Le Bihan, 2007; Osterle & Hammer, 2007). In Italy, where public policies related to long-term care remain underdeveloped, the most important policy measure, both in terms of spending and of people who have access to it, is the Indennità di Accompagnamento (Companionship Payment) (Gori & Da Roit, 2007). In 2008 Israel introduced a pilot program for cash benefit that was further expanded in 2010, whereas England, where direct cash payments have been in place since 1997, started experimentation in 2010 with a pilot program of personal budgets (OECD, 2011). In 2000, Japan implemented a mandatory social insurance program that covers all citizens over the age of 65 years and those between the ages of 40 and 64 years who are affected by an age-related disability (Smiley, 2013, p. 40). A similar approach is to be found in Germany where in 1995/1996 the government introduced the Long-Term Care Insurance Program, a universal and centralized long-term care scheme providing support in cases of care dependency (Theobald & Hampel, 2013).

In the United States, "Cash and Counseling," a nontraditional Medicaid program pioneered by 15 different states, offers the elderly and people with disabilities (NRCPDS website[6])

> . . . the option to manage a flexible budget and decide what mix of goods and services best meet their personal care needs. Participants may use their budget to hire personal care workers, purchase items and make home modifications that help them live independently.

In addition, the 2010 Affordable Care Act (ACA) has increased financial incentives for states to expand home and community-based long-term services (Reinhard et al., 2010).

The result of these strategies has been a progressive transformation of citizens into consumers, a process common in the age of globalization, where health and care are no longer exclusively a citizen's right, but become commodities that can be purchased in the marketplace (Clarke, Newman, Smith, Vidler & Westmarland, 2007; Loyd, 2010). In this landscape, elderly and disabled people are no longer passive objects of care in the hands of the state, but are increasingly construed as individual consumers with spending power who have choices on how to manage chronic and long-term disabilities. Together with the freedom associated with the notion of choice, however, also comes responsibility; care-dependent people and their families become responsible for buying, managing, and organizing their own care. As Foucault explained in his discussion of *governmentality*, the welfare state no longer provides for its citizens directly, but instead becomes a manager and a *trait d'union* between the individual and the market (Foucault, 1991; Gutierrez-Rodriguez, 2011). In other words, the welfare state creates the framework, and families, without being aware of it, enact it. This new role of the welfare state is sometimes quite evident, as in the cash-for-care schemes discussed above, and at other times less so, as in the case of countries such as Italy where the state acts in more indirect ways, such as legislating immigration policies and laws that allow for the creation of a reserve army of labor to supply the increased demand for home eldercare assistance (Degiuli, 2011).

Whereas the introduction of cash-for-care programs in various forms has been adopted in many countries of the Global North, there are variations in the freedom that beneficiaries have in how to spend the funds. While countries such as Italy and Austria, and to a lesser extent Spain and Germany, allow beneficiaries of cash-for-care programs a relatively high degree of freedom, Scandinavian countries and Japan tend to control more closely how funds are spent, the latter actively encouraging in-kind services through its insurance scheme (Lloyd, 2010). Other countries fall in the middle, allowing cash-for-care allowance expenses to be chosen by the beneficiaries, but needing to be approved by social workers (Pavolini & Ranci, 2013). Despite the degree of variation in the freedom associated with cash-for-care programs, a common trend among these countries has been the emergence of private markets of care. These markets entail the increasing presence of private-for-profit and not-for-profit organizations involved in selecting personnel, providing and managing services, and sometimes offering short-term residential care as a respite to family caregivers. In addition to these organizations, there has also been an increase in the number of people independently offering services as home eldercare aids. In many countries this growing labor market relies on immigrant workers. In fact, although the growing marketization of care supposedly provides dependents with more choices and control of the conditions of their care, often the cash allowances, direct payments, or insurance payments offered by various welfare states are not enough to cover the cost of long-term care. When that deficit is coupled with limited control over the spending of these monies, the result is that families tend to hire low-wage careworkers often in the informal labor market (Knijn, 2001).

Although one of the goals of the cash-for-care programs was to address the growing presence of women in the labor market, in reality the increasing reliance on these programs has pushed care back into the hands of families. Instead of finding societal solutions for care and starting a public discussion on eldercare, many welfare states have chosen to defer the provision of services to the consumer marketplace, and to pass the burden to obtain, manage, and maintain care on to individual consumers. The result is that carework, no longer in terms necessarily of provision but in terms of management, ends up in the hands of women because, as many studies show, care continues to be considered for the most part a "women's affair" (Brennan & Williams, 2012; Gutierrez-Rodriguez,

2010). Hence, the organization of care for the elderly ends up increasingly based on individual arrangements managed by private households through informal labor relations, in terms defined by a managerial welfare state. These arrangements often rely on the growing presence and availability of immigrant workers, most often women, in a precarious situation vis-à-vis immigration laws and policies. These workers are highly sought after because together with lower wages, they offer greater flexibility in terms of hours, working conditions, living arrangements, and cultural practices of care. The result is a process of labor outsourcing very common in the contemporary dynamics of globalization; the only difference being that, instead of involving the exporting of manufacturing and services, care outsourcing relies on the importation of people.

CONCLUSIONS

In this chapter I have highlighted how the progressive aging of the population at the world level is generating a language of crisis. Countries are increasingly concerned with how to cope with this impending crisis that will affect them demographically, culturally, economically, and socially. One of the main concerns related to aging has been the increased need for long-term care. In fact, although the majority of citizens in the Global North tend to live longer lives than others, they do not always do that in full health; longer life spans often correspond to longer periods of dependency. In addition to the growing numbers of aging elders requiring higher spending and a larger volume of service, the traditional provision of long-term care is also threatened by demographic, social, and cultural changes such as increased female labor market participation, changes in family structure, intensified mobility, and a decrease in the numbers of women available to care for parents and relatives. To respond to this growing issue, many welfare states of the Global North have introduced market-oriented ideologies and mechanisms to eldercare provision. The result has been a shift in how care for elders is approached, leading to a growing number of cash-for-care programs. Since the introduction of these programs, societies of the Global North have seen parallel developments: on the one hand an increase in the number of formal organizations that provide eldercare services, and on the other an increase in the number of immigrant workers who enter into individual arrangements with private households. The prevalence of one pattern over the other varies from state to state depending on a delicate balance between care regimes and migration regimes.

In either case, by transforming eldercare into a commodity the welfare states of the Global North are implementing a new societal understanding of care, one that reflects neoliberal notions regarding the role of the state, of the market, and of individuals. In the process, care is transformed and so are the experiences and relationships of the main actors who participate in it: from the elders to their families, to the immigrant workers hired to care for them. This transformation, which extends from macrolevel processes such as international migration to microlevel ones such as gender role renegotiation in relationships of care, will be at the core of this book. In the next chapter I focus on the global processes that have allowed for the growing presence of im/migrant workers in eldercare labor markets by exploring the reasons behind the contemporary *feminization of migration*, the global redistribution of reproductive care, and the growth and expansion of the global care chains. In addition, I explore the extent of immigrant labor in different areas of the Global North, and examine the reasons why in some countries hiring an immigrant home eldercare assistant has become the main form of eldercare provision.

NOTES

1 It is important to note that income alone does not necessarily deliver an increase in life expectancy. The increase is connected also to the presence of other elements often present in high- and middle-income countries such as the presence of social services, a solid state-provided infrastructure, political stability, and access to better nutrition. For more information on this please see Biciunate's 2014 article "Economic Growth and Life Expectancy. Do Wealthier Countries Live Longer".

2 The Global Burden of Disease, Injuries, and Risk Factors Study (2010).

3 The increased labor force participation during the past century is especially true of white middle class women, because, as much research has shown, poor and working class women, who were often immigrants and minorities, were already part of the labor market, often informally (see, for example, Amott & Matthei, 1996; Padavic & Reskin, 2002).

Comparing the labor force participation rates for married women from different origin groups is instructive: in 1920 only 7% of married European-American women were in the labor force, compared to 18% of married Asian-American women and one-third of married African-American women (Padavic & Reskin, 2002).

4 In Spain, for example, the rate of women's employment went from 27% in 1981 to 52%, in 2014, in the Netherlands it grew from 36% in 1981 to 68% in 2014, while in Sweden it decreased one percent point from 1981 to 2014 (OECD, 2015).

5 Glazer (1993, p. xi) uses the labor process concept of work transfer or "the shift of tasks from a paid worker to an unpaid family member" to bridge the gap between studies of the labor process and studies of household production.

6 The acronym NRCPDS stands for The National Resource Center for Participant-Directed Services.

2

THE NEW FACES OF ELDERCARE

Strolling along the streets not only of global cities such as New York, Rome, or Sidney, but also of mid-sized cities, towns, and villages of the Global North, it is becoming increasingly common to see aging men and women accompanied in their daily activities by im/migrant women. These couples often capture our attention because in many places they were, until one or two decades ago, an unfamiliar sight. In the past, elderly people in many societies were either institutionalized or assisted by family caregivers, who often looked just like them. Today these couples are eye-catching because they reflect new realities in contemporary societies: the people walking with the elderly of Germany, Spain, and Canada are very often people of different nationalities, ethnicities, religions, and races. These couples have emerged as a result of the trends that I have outlined in the previous chapter, such as aging populations, a progressive decrease in the ability of families to provide care, and a restructuring of welfare states that introduced market-based approaches to the new need for eldercare. They are also the result, however, of other important global trends such as growing income inequality, changes in gender roles, and political and economic developments that have helped to increase and accelerate migration. In other words, as many scholars have pointed out, reproduction and the work connected to it is no longer a national matter, but has become, like production, part of the global economy (among others Anderson, 2000; Chang, 2000; Constable, 1997; Hondagneu Sotelo, 2001; Lan, 2006; Lutz, 2008; Parreñas, 2001; Williams, 2005). Therefore, to understand the current configuration of care provision in many countries of the Global North, together with national welfare state policies, care regimes, and migratory policies, it is crucial to analyze contemporary global and regional migration patterns and trends, global and regional

> political economic developments, regional migratory agreements, and last but not least, sending-countries' strategies for development. In addition, because all of these developments are not neutral but gendered as well as racialized and classed, it is important to explore how these different axes of inequality play a part in shaping current national care arrangements (Kilkey et al., 2010; Lutz, 2008; Williams & Gavanas, 2008).

In this chapter I explore some of the processes that bring im/migrant workers, particularly women, to become a growing and central presence in the provision of eldercare in the Global North. Their presence not only provides support to the women and families of wealthy, postindustrial nations, but also supplies a quick-fix solution for those same welfare states that, due to their presence, are thus able to avoid implementing reforms to deal with the increased need for eldercare. The increased importance of global processes, in fact, should not distract us from the fact that nation-states are still relevant and powerful in defining important areas of social life such as the delivery of welfare, border control, or economic development. In fact, I would argue that nation-states in the contemporary political and economic landscape have not been completely subsumed by supranational organizations, but rather have learned how to work inside the new parameters established by neoliberal restructuring by taking advantage of some of the developments that such restructuring has unchained.

MIGRANT WORKERS MEET FAMILY CAREGIVERS

As highlighted in the previous chapter, the demand for formal and informal eldercare in recent years has been increasing just as the sources of unpaid care at home have been most under pressure. It is important to consider that unpaid care continues to be the most common form of care provided to the aging care-dependent population throughout the world. This is also true of countries of the Global North where, independent of the level of presence or development of the welfare system, families are expected to provide unpaid care both at the beginning and the end of the life cycle (Gooberman-Hill & Ebrahim, 2006). According to Saltman, Rico, and Boerma (2006), the percentage of people relying on family care in Europe continues to be high, reaching peaks of 80% in countries such as Spain, Italy, and Austria, but it is also increasing in countries with stronger welfare states such as Sweden (Lloyd, 2012).

In the United States, family caregivers provide a great deal of unpaid care as well. Economists Kim and Antonopolous (2011) report that according to the 2009 "Caregiving in the U.S." survey:

> An estimated 36.5 million out of 112.6 million households have at least one unpaid family caregiver within the last twelve months. . . The survey

reveals that women (66 percent) are predominantly caregivers with an average age of 48 years old, caring for people over 50 years old (72 percent of care receivers). On average, caregiving has been ongoing for 4.6 years; 31 percent of caregivers have been caring for their loved ones for five years or more. The caregivers spend 20.4 hours a week on average, with 26 percent spending over 20 hours a week. The burden of care, measured by care time and number of care activities regarding daily living, is high for 32 percent of caregivers.

Together with highlighting the role of family caregivers in the provision of care, the above quote also highlights the fact that long-term care continues to be, for the most part, the responsibility of women (Marchetti, 2015; U.S. Bureau of Labor Statistics, 2015a). This is true not only for the United States but for the majority of countries of the Global North. The analysis of data concerning 17 different OECD countries, in fact, shows that women account for close to two-thirds of all caregivers aged 50 to 75 years (Figure 2.1).

Whereas the data cited above show that overall intergenerational support mechanisms remain strong, studies also show that family caregivers often struggle to maintain a balance between the demands of care and those of work.

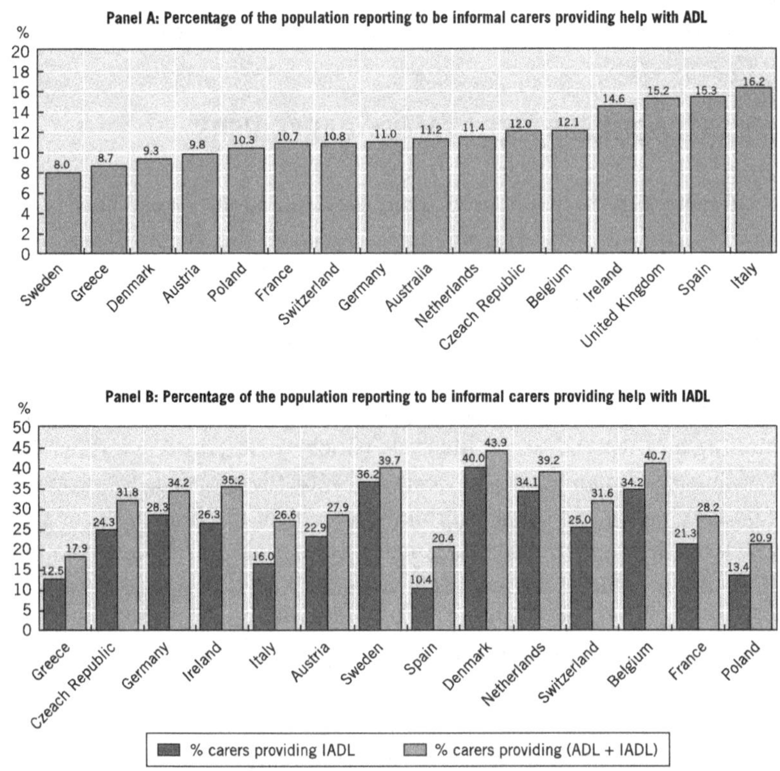

Figure 2.1. Caregiving by European country and type of support provided to the elders. *Source:* OECD (Colombo et al. 2011, p.69).

Long-term care for the elders, in fact, tends to increase over time, extending its demands often into hours usually dedicated to family and work life. Studies show that family members providing unpaid care often are less likely to be involved in the formal labor market and/or to be involved in full-time work, particularly when the hours of care increase over time (Carmichael & Charles, 2003; Heitmueller, 2007; Viitanen, 2005). According to the OECD study, *Help Wanted. Providing and Paying for Long-Term Care* (2011), the more hours a family caregiver provides, the more likely that she or he will give up outside employment, especially when the amount of care required goes beyond 20 hours a week. The needs related to eldercare provision also affect family caregivers' career choices, and in many cases the wages that they can secure for themselves. Caregivers, in fact, often experience a wage penalty due to career interruption, deterioration of human capital, skill depreciation, and the lack of advancement opportunity (Earle & Heymann, 2011). Because of these difficulties, family caregivers of working age can find themselves at a higher risk for poverty, and this is particularly true for women, especially when they are single (OECD, 2011). For these reasons, most family caregivers at some point or another try to find support and assistance for their care provision. Although most welfare states acknowledge the need to provide support to family caregivers—not necessarily because care is considered an important element of societal reproduction, but because encouraging women to enter the labor market is a key policy in reducing overall welfare spending—this support tends to translate into cash provision rather than actual services. In addition, welfare support is often provided only to the most economically vulnerable sector of the population, leaving all other family caregivers struggling. The result is more pressure for family caregivers who not only have to provide some level of care, but also, in many cases, have to organize, manage, and secure eldercare for long periods of time and often for more than one elder at a time. In some countries, such as England, Japan, and the United States, this increased need for eldercare support can be satisfied through the formal care labor market, due to the presence of multiple private agencies offering this kind of support. In many other countries, such as Germany, Italy, and Spain, the informal labor market remains the quickest, cheapest, and most flexible way to obtain help. This is why in many countries of the Global North eldercare is increasingly shared or completely outsourced to im/migrant women, often of color[1] (see, among others Bettio, Simonazzi, & Villa, 2006; Da Roit, 2010; Degiuli, 2007; van Hooren, 2014), or, as in the case of the United States, a combination of immigrant and minority women (Boris & Klein, 2012; Browne & Braun, 2008; Stacey, 2011). Women, in fact, continue to be the workers of choice in the long-term care sector mostly due to gender stereotypes and cultural norms that continue to portray women as *naturally* able to care. These gender notions are often coupled with idealized notions of race and ethnicity, ranking some groups as more *prone* to care than others, thereby creating an imagined workforce whose ability to provide care is thought to surpass that of other people.

Racial and ethnic minority women and immigrants, as noted by Glenn (1992, 2010), have met domestic and carework needs for many decades, yet the increased mobility of workers across the world has exacerbated both the global and regional nature of these processes. The creation of labor markets of care, in fact, is not determined only by household and individual needs, but is also the result of other changes such as: new immigration patterns, global and regional political and economic developments, and nation-state-based migration policies in both sending and receiving countries. In the next section I will review some of the policies and ideologies enforced both at the global and national level that have increased the availability of im/migrant women in the care labor markets of the Global North—an availability that has not diminished even after the economic recession started in 2008 (Kilkey, Perrons, & Plomien, 2013).

THE FEMINIZATION OF MIGRATION

One of the most striking trends of the past 30 years in migration has been what scholars and policy makers have called the *feminization of migration*. According to the International Organization for Migration (2013), "The total number of international migrants has increased from an estimated 150 million in 2000 to 214 million persons today." Women constitute roughly half of all international im/migrants worldwide (UN DESA PD, 2013) and they tend to concentrate, as shown in Figure 2.2, in wealthier areas of the world, namely North America, Europe, East Asia, Australia, and the Middle East, where they take on significant amounts of domestic work, childcare, and,

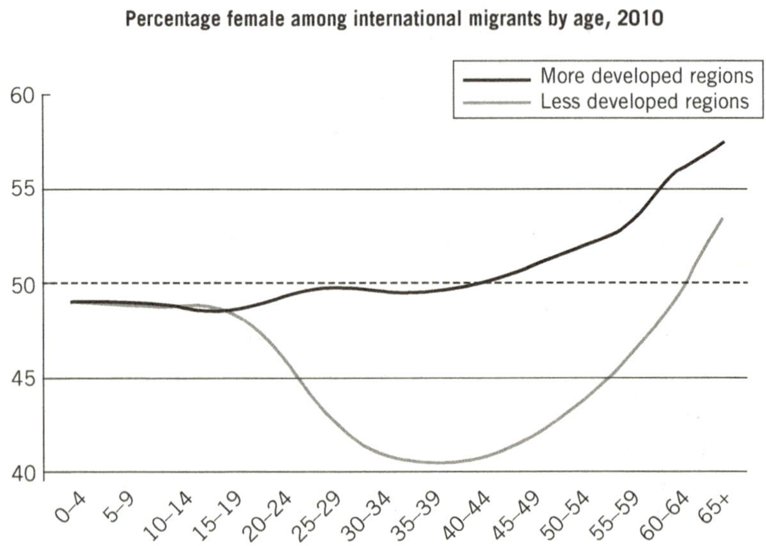

Figure 2.2. Percentage of female international migrants by age 2010. *Source:* United Nations Department of Economic and Social Affairs Population Division (2012) *The Age and Sex of Migrants*. Available at http://www.un.org/en/development/desa/population/publications/pdf/migration/age-sex-migrants-wallchart_2011.pdf.

increasingly eldercare, thus generating what Parreñas (2001) has termed the new *international division of reproductive labor.* Italy, in this sense, provides a vantage point for the observation of this phenomenon because women have represented more than half of the migratory fluxes in the country for the past 10 years and are now the majority among the im/migrant resident population (Agostini, C., Longobardi, E., & Vitaletti, G. 2012). In addition, immigration in Italy for the purpose of domestic work is not necessarily a recent development but one that started, albeit in slightly different form, in the 1970s (Andall, 2000; Tognetti-Bordogna, 2012).

EXPLAINING GENDERED IMMIGRATION PATTERNS

Neoclassical economic theory tends to explain immigration patterns by focusing on im/migrants' choices based on elements such as unemployment and low wages (Massey, Arango, Hugo, Kouaouci, Pellegrino, & Taylor, 1998; Misra, Woodring, & Merz, 2006). Contrary to this theory, recent studies on care and domestic work focus on globalization processes and their role in creating and reproducing a reserve army of women workers (Anderson, 2000; Chang, 2000; Ehrenreich & Hochschild, 2002; Parreñas, 2001; Pyle & Ward, 2003). Since the 1970s, changes in the global political economy have had a dramatic effect on the lives of women, who have become increasingly integrated as active participants in both production and consumption processes (Enloe, 1990, 2000; Freeman, 2000; Marchand & Runyan, 2010; Mills, 1999; Pyle &Ward, 2003). A theoretical framework that helps to understand these developments has been developed over time by sociologist Saskia Sassen (1984, 1988, 1999, 2001, 2004), who suggests that globalization requires the cheap labor of women in the export processing zones of the countries of the Global South and also in what is left of manufacturing and service sectors in countries of the Global North. (Parreñas, 2006). As a result of gendered expectations, women have become the workforce of choice in this political, economic, and cultural environment. Employers, in fact, perceive women as easier to control, less demanding in terms of rights and wages, and, often, easier to dismiss than men. In addition, they are considered more apt, as an extension of their biological make-up, to provide care for the children and the elderly and to perform domestic work.

In her books Sassen outlines two different economic trends impacting global labor markets. The first is the increasingly high mobility of capital, which has made accumulation on a world scale possible to an unprecedented degree. Such mobility has been actively encouraged by supranational institutions such as the International Monetary Fund (IMF) and the World Bank, which, through the implementation of structural adjustment programs, have pressured countries across the Global South to adopt neoliberal economic policies by reducing tariffs and trade barriers and opening their financial markets (Robinson, 2007). The progressive disappearance of barriers to the mobility of capital has been matched by technological and social innovations, which have created a compression of space and time that in turn has made it possible for companies to move production rapidly from one place to another (Castells, 1996). Both of these changes have had immense consequences for the global labor market in terms of both location and compensation (Standing, 1999). As capital has become increasingly able to operate on this global scale, huge reserves of cheap labor have been drawn from all over the world into increasingly centralized systems of production (Castles & Miller, 2003). This increased need for labor has often pushed employers and/or their agents to tap into the subsistence sectors of the Global South, uprooting people, particularly young women, from existing economic and social systems, transforming them into migrants. (Massey, Durand, & Malone, 2005; Parreñas, 2001; Sassen, 1999).

The displacement of workers linked to the transformation of production across the world was then matched, according to Sassen (1991/2001), by a second trend: that of a reorganization of the labor market in postindustrial societies. If the process outlined above tends to create migrants and transform them into low-wage workers, the second, instead, is geared to absorb them once they arrive in the wealthy, post-industrial countries of the Global North (Parreñas, 2001). As industrial production has moved overseas, the traditional manufacturing industries in countries of the Global North have almost disappeared and been partially replaced by a downgraded, deskilled manufacturing sector characterized by poorly paid jobs and accompanied by a rapid growth of the service sector. This sector includes companies specializing in finance, accounting, insurance, advertising, marketing, and research and design that have been growing in major European and American cities since the 1980s and 1990s due to the need for multinational corporations to concentrate their operations in global nodes (Sassen, 1991/2001). The concentration of flexible, highly paid professionals in major cities in turn requires the presence of low-wage service workers to help them reproduce and maintain their lifestyles. These service-oriented jobs include restaurant workers, caterers, domestic workers, spa and nail salon workers, nannies, dog walkers, and errand runners, among others. (Robinson, 2009, pp. 15–16). Remarkably, many of the low paying jobs created in the Global North are highly gendered both because these jobs are often considered *women's jobs* and because their wages and conditions are so poor that only *secondary breadwinners* are likely to accept them (Standing, 2001).[2] Consequently, many of the im/migrants who respond to the increasing demand for low-wage workers in these countries were, and continue to be, women (Misra, Woodring, & Merz, 2006; Parreñas, 2001; Sassen, 1991/2001).

Global economic and political transformations, however, were not the only reasons behind contemporary migratory fluxes; regional transformations also played a part in generating migration flows. The collapse of the Soviet Union in 1991 and the transition from socialist to free market economies, as well as the Russian economic, currency, and financial crisis of the late 1990s, generated extensive migratory movements first from countries such as Poland, Romania, Albania, and the former Yugoslavia and then from areas such as Moldova, Ukraine, Lithuania, and Estonia (Kofman et al., 2000; Tognetti-Bordogna, 2012).

These developments taken together have generated the trend, mentioned above, known as "feminization of migration." This trend does not necessarily refer to the number of women migrating both regionally and globally, because women have been migrating alongside men in high numbers since the 1960s, but rather to a qualitative change in the migratory experience (Zlotnik, 2003). Today women no longer migrate only as *secondary migrants* to follow the males of the family, rather they do so as *primary migrants*, starting their own migratory project alone and, often, leaving their families behind. They do not necessarily choose that pattern, but host countries often make it difficult for their children and partners/spouses to travel with them (Lutz, 2011).

The changes in the global economy of the 1980s and 1990s described above also generated many of the political, economic, and cultural shifts discussed in Chapter 1, including increased participation of women in the labor market, growing mobility, and the progressive demise of extended families, which have increased the demand for domestic and care labor. The result is that the demand for im/migrant women's labor has expanded beyond global cities to become capillary and central also to smaller cities, towns, and villages of Europe, North America, parts of Asia, and the oil-rich countries of the Middle East. This demand has created an ever-growing care labor market and generated what Arlie Hochschild has defined as the *global care chain* whereby women from the Global South seek employment outside their countries providing care and domestic support to families of the Global North, while leaving their own children and families to be cared for by other women (Hochschild, 2000). In addition, it has also spurred the migration of older women, particularly from the Russian Federation and Eastern Europe, who through circular migration can continue to support the rebuilding of their nations (Solari, 2011).

The increasing availability of women in the global labor market. However, has not simply been the result of increased demand for domestic and care work, but has also been supported by the effects of structural adjustment programs implemented by the IMF and the World Bank in many countries of the Global South. These programs, aside from implementing free trade and the removal of barriers for capital, also required countries of the above mentioned areas to increasingly deregulate, privatize, reduce social spending, and devalue the local currency in exchange for loans (Chang, 2000; Lindio-McGovern, 2012; Sassen, 2004). Such policies, although ideally aimed at "balancing the budget" and integrating countries into the global economy, in reality, had sizable negative effects on the daily livelihood of the poor in the Global South, and particularly poor women. Sadasivam (1997), chief of the Civil Society Team at the United Nations Population Division (UNPD), argues that although the language of structural adjustment programs (SAP) is alleged to be gender-neutral, it has a male bias and the use of gender-neutral economic terms masks the reality of a gendered division of labor. For example, even though SAPs require states to reduce or eliminate many social programs and subsidies with damaging consequences on entire communities, the gendered effects vary substantially. Sadasivam (1997, p. 632) writes, "Austerity . . . is a female responsibility: men tend to maintain their social and personal expenditures, while women are expected to make ends meet with fewer resources, by working longer hours within and outside the home." This statement is supported by multiple studies conducted in the past 25 years that show that the IMF and World Bank's programs often rely upon the ability of individual families, and specifically women, to compensate for the loss of state-funded social services (among others: Beneria & Feldman 1992; Bergeron, 2001; Harrison, 1997; Susser, 1997).

Deregulation, another key requirement of SAPs, also has gendered implications. Sociologist Lindio-McGovern (2012, p. 11) argues:

> Deregulation refers to implementing policy measures that dismantle or minimize state regulations of the market, such as price control system of basic commodities, protection of labor rights, environment, wage systems and the practices of corporations. Often deregulation hurts most the poor, the low-income families and consumers, indigenous communities, low-wage workers, and the unemployed.

Because women are the majority of these segments of the population the overall result is that women increasingly find it difficult to provide food for their families, obtain livable wages, and secure a healthy environment for their families and children. Concurrently, the tightened economic conditions that result from SAPs reduce opportunities for formal wage employment and increase dependence on informal means of income provision. It is therefore not a surprise that women often resort to migration in order to provide for their families, and—although they may view their experiences as resulting from private decisions—these decisions are actually a response to governments' needs to balance their trade and pay off their international debt. As Enloe (1989/2000, p. 185) points out:

> When a woman from Mexico, Jamaica, or the Philippines decides to emigrate in order to make money as a domestic worker she is designing her own international debt politics. She is trying to cope with the loss of earning power and the rise in the cost of living at home by cleaning bathrooms in the land of bankers.

The argument Enloe makes goes beyond domestic work and includes all forms of gendered and feminized work that revolves around the provision of care, as well as emotional, and often sex work.

The global dynamics that generate the international division of reproductive labor play out not only at the global level but also at the regional level—a fact that helps to explain more localized movements of women (Kilkey et al., 2013; Sarti, 2008; Williams, 2010). This is the case, for example, for women from Eastern Europe who move to Western and Southern Europe, of Mexican women who move to the United States (Hondagneu Sotelo, 2001), and of Filipino, Thai, and Indonesian women who move to Hong Kong and Taiwan, among other countries (Constable, 2007; Pei Chia Lan, 2006).

Finally, to fully understand contemporary female migration, in addition to the analysis of global labor market transformations and of the role of supranational organizations such as the IMF and the World Bank, it is crucial to explore the role played by neoliberal states both at the receiving and sending end (Castles & Miller, 2003; Portes, 1997). As Parreñas (2001, p. 28) points out, "transnational processes do not supercede, but are embedded in the institution of the nation-state." The analysis of state policies and discourses associated with migration, therefore, provides us with a deeper understanding of how migration processes are generated by political decisions, economic calculations, and cultural notions that, while supporting the neoliberal ideology inherent to the globalization process, are also aimed at solving labor market shortages at the national level (Misra, Woodring, & Merz, 2006; Williams, 2010). Migration policies, in fact, not only shape the scale, characteristics, and experience of im/migrant domestic and care workers as a whole, but also create hierarchies and consequently subjects with different levels of vulnerability in the labor market. This is not a new process, according to Heisler (1985, p. 475):

> Post World-War II European labor migrations were not haphazard result of push and pull factors. Rather they resulted from deliberate policy decisions, were initiated by the host country, and guided by bilateral agreements with the sending country.

Similar processes also characterize the history of migration in the United States and other countries of the Global North where workers are selected on the basis of both national origin and skills to fill specific voids in the labor market (see Filipino nurses in the United States or Cabo Verdian domestic workers in Italy). What has changed today is the extent and acceleration of migrant flows both at the global and regional level, which in turn allow receiving countries to be more selective. Today's hierarchies of labor include women from all corners of the world, with varying levels of education, skill, and abilities, whose migratory projects and working conditions will differ greatly depending, in part, on their ability to secure a proper visa. In the case of Italy, for example, these hierarchies are quite visible. Women migrating from Bulgaria and Romania, though not belonging to the passport free area of the European Union (EU), are able to enter and work legally in the country. This facility of entrance in turn affects both their migratory journey—they have more freedom in choosing the length of their stay in the country—and their employment conditions, because their legal status provides them with stronger bargaining power when dealing with employers. Their experience is countered by that of women from countries as different as Albania, Peru or Nigeria, who, for lack of access to a legal visa, enter the country irregularly. These women tend to choose long-term migratory projects due to their inability to go back and forth, and will most likely be pushed into the most vulnerable positions in the domestic and care market.

In addition, quota systems, guest worker programs, and special visas also allow states of the Global North to refine their selection process and solve local shortages in the labor market in an effective manner. In Italy, for example, the quota system for domestic workers has a long history (Andall, 2000). At its inception it was designed to provide domestic workers for upper-middle-class families and replace the dwindling presence of Italian women in the sector (Sarti, 2013). Over time the goals of the quota have changed to reflect and accommodate the growing needs for care expressed by Italian families of all social classes. This quota system has multiple functions. On the one hand it allows the state to choose and pick the workers needed not only in terms of skills but also indirectly in terms of gender, and on the other it provides the state with a low-cost solution for the historical shortage of welfare services. The introduction of a cheap and vulnerable labor force available to support Italian families has allowed the Italian state to avoid directly engaging in more substantial reform of the welfare state or in a much needed discussion of the value of reproductive labor, both in terms of child and eldercare in Italian society.

Italy is not the only country of the Global North to utilize immigration policies to, not only, solve shortages but also to segment the domestic and care labor market. Similar examples either in the forms of quotas, special visas, or guest worker programs can be found from Germany to the United States, and from Hong Kong to the oil-rich Gulf countries (among others Gutierrez, 2010; Kofman, 2012; Lan, 2006; Näre, 2013; Yeates, 2009).

Receiving states are not the only ones engaged in creating, shaping, and organizing migratory flows; sending countries increasingly play an important role in this as well. Remittances, the money sent home from international migrants, have, in recent decades, become for many countries of Eastern Europe and the Global South one of the most important and most resilient economic sources, even more important than foreign direct investment, overseas aid, and private loans (Sirkeci, Cohen, & Ratha, 2012). According to Sirkeci, Cohen and Ratha (2012, p. 2): "Remittance flows to developing countries totaled about $75 billion in 1989, $125 billion by the mid-2000s, and more than $350 billion by 2011 despite about a 5 percent decline in 2009."

This constant flow of money is crucial for sending countries because, among other things, it ensures a range of investments that contributes to the gross domestic product (GDP) by supporting consumption, small enterprises, and capital investments that improve local livelihoods (Bach, 2011, p. 131). Remittances are not a new phenomenon per se—migrants have sent money home to their families for centuries—what is new, however, is the increased attention that government institutions, international financial organizations, nongovernmental organizations (NGOs), and the overall development community are paying to them and to their potential for poverty reduction (Bach, 2011; Kunz, 2011). This new understanding of the role of remittances has generated a new approach from all these different organizations that are now concentrating on how to harness their potential. Sending states, in particular, are becoming more and more involved in shaping, organizing, and managing the migration of their own citizens. They do this in a variety of ways: by creating programs that help to speed up the *authorization* workers need to travel abroad, by training workers to acquire the skills requested by receiving countries, and by developing *ideological* discourses to ensure that migrants remain tightly connected to their countries of origin.

An example of these different processes is provided by sociologist Robyn Rodriguez in her book *Migrants for Exports* (2010), in which she explores the role of the Philippine state in facilitating outward migration of its own citizens. As mentioned in the previous section, countries of the Global North have become increasingly selective in allowing im/migrants into their territory. Thus, authorization to enter the countries of the Global North has become increasingly difficult to obtain and requires extensive knowledge of migration policies in different countries on the one hand, and particular skills and abilities that allow migrants to obtain special visa status, enter guest worker programs, or apply through different quota systems on the other. Keenly aware of these barriers, the Philippine state has created agencies that help Philippine nationals to obtain the highly desirable *authorized status*. The state has devised a double-pronged approach to addressing this issue. First, it has created two agencies, the Philippine Overseas Employment Administration (POEA) and the International Labor Affairs Service (ILAS), whose aim is to monitor trends in labor demand globally, while at the same time paying close attention to immigration policies. The agencies are also supported by the Philippines' diplomatic corps that conducts overall labor market research, identifies employment trends, and also initiates conversations with potential receiving countries to facilitate the entrance of Philippine workers into specific labor markets (Rodriguez, 2010, p. 24).

The state complements its research and brokerage by providing training to help migrants acquire the skills needed in a diverse labor market. To achieve this goal the Philippine state ensures training through the Technical Education and Skills Development Authority (TESDA). This agency, which trains workers both for international and national employment, first makes sure that Philippine workers are familiar with English, then selects and licenses private facilities to train workers in the areas and skills required by global labor demands (Lorente, 2011; Rodriguez, 2010).

Although the Philippine state system of labor brokerage is quite sophisticated compared to that of other countries and in many cases helps to strengthen the status of Philippine migrant workers around the world (Philippine women workers are usually at the top of the hierarchy in domestic and care labor in many countries to the point of being dubbed "the Mercedes Benz of domestic workers"), other sending states also provide training to make their migrant workers more acceptable to receiving countries. Sri Lanka, for example, is beginning to offer training for domestic workers going to Saudi Arabia, and is planning to extend the program in to workers going to other West Asian countries (http://www.colombopage.com/archive_13B/Jul14_1373820640JR.php). Whereas the Sri Lankan program has emerged partially in response to growing reports of abuse toward domestic workers and in response to the adoption by the International Labor Organization on June 2011 of a groundbreaking treaty that extends key labor protections, it is also aimed at "professionalizing" migrant women in order to secure higher wages and consequently higher remittances (http://www.arabnews.com/news/464014).

In addition to supporting outward migration through brokering and "professionalization," sending countries also actively attempt to channel and augment remittances in order to leverage development. Economist Sarah Gammage (2006, p. 7) looks at the specific case of El Salvador and explains:

> Government-sponsored programs are being developed and refined to capture these remittances and focus their expenditure through co-financing. Agencies such as the Fondo de Inversion Social para el Desarrollo Local (Social Investment Fund for Local Development–FISDL) offer co-financing to Salvadoran communities and hometown associations to invest their collective remittances. The government is also actively reaching out to communities of Salvadorans abroad through its embassies and cultural services to stimulate interest in investing individual and collective remittances and recruit economic and philanthropic projects.

The practices highlighted by Gammage are not unique to El Salvador; instead they have become common practice among sending countries of the Global South and Eastern Europe, due also to the encouragement received by the World Bank, the Inter American Development Bank, the IMF, and other supranational institutions concerned with development. These organizations, in fact, are quite vocal in pushing government to create programs aimed at channeling individual and collective remittances. And although all migrants are targeted through these policies, states tend to pay particular attention to women migrants who have been identified from the development community as more reliable and constant in their remittances (Bach, 2011).

CONCLUSIONS

The analysis of all the different actors involved in creating, shaping, and managing migration flows shows that the supply and demand model, often used to understand the growing presence of im/migrant women in the labor markets of care in the Global North, is not sufficient to explain the complexity and contradictions inherent to contemporary labor migration. Contemporary labor migrants, particularly women migrants, are often portrayed in public discourse as people in need coming to the Global North looking for a better life. These assertions are often too simplistic and tend to hide the fact the im/migrant women are actually the back upon which the reality of neoliberal thinking is built. Im/migrant women are displaced from their community of origin because of global labor restructuring, political and economic crisis, and policies implemented by supranational organizations such as the IMF, the World Bank, and the World Trade Organization (WTO), which have enforced policies that helped to dismantle local industries, reduce state-based services, and limit the quality and quantity of jobs available. In the process, women enter migration circuits in which they shoulder the cost of rich countries' unwillingness to respond with public, state-based solutions to the growing needs for reproductive care in the Global North. Furthermore, in addition to providing economic support to their families and communities, they are also central to national strategies of economic growth in many countries of the Global South, and of national political and economic rebuilding in many countries of Eastern Europe. The mobilization of im/migrant women across the world therefore serves multiple functions at the local and global level, none of which is usually made visible to the societies that receive them. In addition, their mobilization and their work are crucial in masking the shortcomings of ideologies and practices that tend to individualize the responsibility of reproductive work instead of recognizing its collective importance and the responsibility all societies have to provide care for their populations.

NOTES

1 Research shows that there are also some men employed in this labor market, and although this constitutes a very important development, the majority of immigrant workers employed as *home eldercare assistants* continue to be

women. For this reason from now on I will refer exclusively to immigrant women when talking about the workers involved in this occupation.

2 This refers to what Guy Standing (2001) has defined as the feminization of labor, whereby not only is there an increasing number of women in the labor market, but the current working conditions are similar to the ones usually associated with women's jobs: part-time, no benefits, temporary, and so on.

3

THE ITALIAN CASE

> Every time I return to Italy from California I am surprised to see how things have changed. When I left in 1996, immigration in Turin, Italy was already something we talked about . . . the Moroccans in Porta Palazzo, the Albanians in piazza Carducci, but it was definitely still something distant, not quite real; there was definitely an "us versus them" sense and things still looked temporary, as if these newcomers could still disappear at any moment. Today things look different . . . everywhere I go I encounter these odd looking couples: young, tall energetic African women pushing frail Italian elders on wheelchairs, Peruvian middle-aged women and elderly Italian men and women shopping together at the local supermarkets, and at the park it is increasingly common to see on one bench three elderly Italian women basking in the sun and chatting, while their Filipino caregivers are doing the same on the nearby bench. And, in some cases, there is a strong sense of intimacy in these couples; on the surface these women do not seem to appear as "others," they seem to be very much part of everyday reality, just like the bakery at the corner or the tobacconist in the neighborhood square. When did this happen? What made it happen? And most importantly is it true that their position vis-à-vis Italian society has changed? (Field notes May 5, 2002.)

In the previous chapters I outlined the increasing need for long-term elder-care assistance that is emerging at the global level while situating it at the convergence of a number of trends including the aging of the population, changes in labor market structure and participation, shifts in family structure, and a restructuring of the welfare state. As a result of these developments, an increasing number of services have been removed from the household and converted into paid services to be purchased in the marketplace. This transfer has, over the years, come to match another growing trend explored in Chapter 2, the increased presence of women in migratory movements across the world, a presence generated by political–economic and cultural transformations both at the global and local level that dislocate women from their countries of origin and channel them into the low-wage service sectors of wealthier societies, particularly into the care and domestic sector. In this chapter I will highlight how these global structural changes become embedded in the political, economic, and cultural specificity of the local society, in this case Italy, generating new realities and new forms of social organizations. Scholars of globalization, in fact, have pointed out that what we call globalization is not a "thing" that floats above us; rather it is the result of a set of processes that are actually produced on the ground in local context by specific social actors including institutions, nongovernmental organizations (NGOs), and private individuals (Buroway, 2000; Solari, 2014: 134). Italy, in this sense, offers an excellent case study to explore these assertions because it provides us with the opportunity to see how these macroscale processes ground themselves in the reality of everyday lives. The developments described in Chapter 1 have found very fertile ground in Italy: a country with one of the oldest populations in the world, in which demographic, economic, and cultural transformations together with changes in labor market participation have affected the institution of the family and its ability to provide unpaid care, and an obsolete familialist[1] welfare state is struggling to address these ongoing transformations. In this context, when families are consistently struggling under multiple care needs, the growing presence of im/migrant women has come to represent a flexible and available market solution to many of their problems. So much so that temporary solutions have been transformed into a central element of the contemporary organization of long-term care (Lippi Bruno & Ugolini, 2013). The National Institute of Social Security, for example, reports that the number of im/migrant women legally employed in the domestic sector grew by 74% between 2002 and 2011, to stand at nearly 766,000 regular workers (Barbiano Di Belgioso & Ortensi, 2013; INPS, 2013). The Italian Institute for Statistical Studies, instead, mindful of the fact that many of these working relations take place in the gray area of the informal labor market, estimates that in 2013 the number of people employed in domestic and care-related services was actually closer to 1,665,000. Although the total number of domestic and care workers may remain impossible to determine, a study conducted by Censis and ISMU in 2013 that included a sample of 1,500 workers in Italy provides a useful snapshot of the geographic distribution of these workers (Table 3.1), their gender, and their overall age.

Table 3.1 shows that the domestic and care labor market is composed largely of women between the ages of 36 and 50 years who are predominantly foreigners. In fact, even though the data show an Italian presence among these workers, the majority continues to remain foreigners. Foreigners account respectively for 81.4% and 81.7% in the North and Center of Italy and for 64.3% in Southern

Table 3.1. Geographic Distribution of Domestic and Care Workers

	Geographic Area			
	North	**Center**	**South**	**Total**
Nationality				
Italians	18.6	18.3	35.7	22.7
Foreigners	81.4	81.7	64.3	77.3
Total	100.0	100.0	100.0	100.0
Sex				
Female	81.8	83.3	82.5	82.4
Male	18.2	16.7	17.5	17.6
Total	100.0	100.0	100.0	100.0
Age				
From 18 to 35	22.9	24.3	26.2	24.1
36–50	57.3	56.5	56.3	56.8
50 and over	19.8	19.2	17.5	19.1
Total	100.0	100.0	100.0	100.0

Source: Censis-ISMU (2013).

Italy where the presence of Italian workers becomes more significant (35.7) but still well below that of foreign workers (Censis & ISMU, 2013).

In the following sections I will explore in depth some of the above-mentioned developments and their intersections to explain how the current arrangements of long-term care in Italy came into place.

ITALY IS AN OLD COUNTRY

One of the main characteristics of the Italian population is its age. While Italy has recently lost the primacy of the oldest population of the world to Japan and Germany (Hayutin, 2010), its population remains one of the oldest of the world with a median age of 43.3 years and an aging index of 147.2[2] (ISTAT, 2013a). The aging of the population in Italy started almost 50 years ago, right after the 1960s baby boom years, when the country began to undergo changes in social and cultural practices, lifestyles, and behaviors (Mazza & Capacci, 2006). As in the case of many industrialized nations, the contemporary age structure of the Italian population is the result of a reduction in mortality rates combined with a substantial drop in fertility rates and a progressive increase in life expectancy for both men and women. The fertility rate in Italy started to drop later than in the rest of Europe, but once it did, it did so quickly; the rate went from 2.43 offspring per woman in the 1970s to 1.19 in 1995[3] (ISTAT, 2005). The stagnation in population growth extended from 1985 to 2001, the year in which the fertility rate began to grow again, albeit moderately, mainly due to migration flows. Although the fertility rate has oscillated between 1.37 and 1.42 in the past decade, the growth has not been large enough to bring the population to a positive balance, which means that the country continues to have more deaths than births on a regular basis (Gagliardi et al., 2012; ISTAT, 2015).

Together with a drop in fertility, Italy has experienced a progressive decrease in mortality and it is now considered one of the countries with the highest longevity. Data for the past 30 years show that the survival rates have been increasing for all age groups. However, it is in the older age groups that the results become striking: at age 65 years, the mortality rates have been halved, dropping in 2007 from 27.9 per thousand in 1974 to 14.5 per thousand for men and from 13.5 to 6.9 per thousand for women. In addition, the overall percentage of the population 65 years and over has grown from 15.1 in 1991 to 20.21 in 2013 (ISTAT, 2007; Ministero del Lavoro e delle Politiche Sociali, 2013). Owing to medical and technological progress and an improvement in socioeconomic conditions year after year, the number of people who reach old age increases; today the overall life expectancy is 84.9 years for women and 80.2 for men (ISTAT, 2015). The decline in mortality rates is also a significant factor in the increase in the proportion of *oldest old* among the elderly population. This group too has grown in numbers going from 2.4% of the population in 1992 to 6.1% in 2013 (Ministero del Lavoro e delle Politiche Sociali, 2013). Overall, according to estimates provided by the Italian Institute for Statistical Studies in 2011, in Italy there were 12.3 million women and men over the age of 65 years and 6.1 million citizens over the age of 75 years (ISTAT, 2013b).

The result of these developments is thus an increase both in the total number of elderly people and in their proportion when compared to other age groups (Buccianti, 2004), a fact that becomes particularly evident when looking at the aging index, an index that compares the proportions of the *young population* (0–14 years) to the *old population* (65 years and over). In Italy at the end of 2011, the last year for which there is available data, there were 148 elderly people for every 100 young people (ISTAT, 2013a), and although the numbers already seem staggering, they are only destined to grow. Joseph Troisi, professor of Social Gerontology and Director of the European Centre for Gerontology at the University of Malta, predicts that the percentage of the aging population in Italy will continue to increase, reaching 34.4% in 2025 and 41.3% in 2050 (Troisi, 2013).

Although the aging of the population is not necessarily a negative development, it certainly has many societal effects, one being the increased need for long-term care and assistance. As mentioned in the Chapter 1, in fact, the increase in life expectancy has not necessarily carried with it the assurance of a better quality of life. According to statistics compiled by Eurostat, only 34% of the population between the ages of 65 and 74 years considers himself or herself to be in good health; this number goes down to 17% among the population 75 to 84 years and it drops to 13% for the population 85 years and over (Eurostat, 2013). The majority of this population is afflicted with at least one chronic disease (55.0% in the group 55–59 years old reaching 86.4% among the population 75 years and over), and often by two at the same time (68.1% of the population 75 years and over) (ISTAT, 2013a). A similar pattern is evident when talking about the limitations in everyday activities.

Although these numbers provide a useful snapshot of the issue, it is important to point out that they do not reveal the actual extent of the problem. Care for elderly people extends well beyond disabled ones. In fact, even when in good health, elderly people need support in a variety of daily activities, in remaining safe, and, in some cases, simply coping with solitude, loneliness, and depression. The aging of the population therefore carries with it an increased need for care and support, a need that often remains invisible and difficult to describe in all its facets.

This increase in need comes at a time when the historical providers of care, namely Italian families, and more specifically the women in those families, are no longer capable of responding to the growing demand. Historically, the care for the young and the elders in Italy has been provided as unpaid reproductive labor by family networks. Numerous studies have shown the crucial role played by both the immediate and the extended family in providing care services that a weak and fragmented welfare state was not able to provide (Da Roit, 2010; Naldini & Saraceno, 2008; Zanatta, 2005). Due to economic, demographic, political, and social transformations, however, Italian families have changed and are no longer able to provide the care that is needed, a situation that is creating growing tensions.

THE TRANSFORMATION OF ITALIAN FAMILIES

To begin, it is important to note that the numbers of Italian women available for care are dwindling. In fact, some of the same demographic trends that have caused the aging of the population, namely a decrease in fertility together with a decrease in family size, have also reduced the number of daughters and daughters-in-law who previously provided the greatest amount of care for elders (Glucksmann & Lyon, 2006; Zanatta, 2005). Therefore, today the increasing requests for care have to be shouldered by a smaller number of people. This situation creates further strain, a strain compounded by a progressive transformation of family structures brought about by socioeconomic, politic, and cultural changes. Families in Italy, and in Southern Europe in general, have changed a great deal over the past 50 years, particularly in the past decade (Naldini & Jurado, 2009). Starting in the 1950s, Italy has experienced a progressive increase in the percentage of the population living in nuclear families and a corresponding decrease in the percentage of extended families. At the beginning of this process, nuclear families were mostly married couples with children; today such families constitute only 36.4% of the total. Italy has also experienced the emergence of new family structures such as single parenthood, cohabitation, and reconstituted families. By 2009 the number of these new family forms had reached almost 7 million, involving 20% of the total population (ISTAT, 2011). Although these transformations do not necessarily hinder intergenerational support as many studies show, they have an impact on the organization of social life and consequently on the ability of families to be the main provider of care (Albert & Ferring, 2013).

A model that has been growing rapidly in recent years has been the single-parent one. Today, single-parent households amount to 15.1% of all nuclear families, compared to 1988 when they were 9.6% (ISTAT, 2003, 2013a). Although this growth does not appear great at first glance, what is relevant is the shift in the reasons that cause it. In 1988, the majority of single-headed households were linked to widowhood or, to a lesser extent, extramarital births, but by 2013 an increasing percentage of these families had been formed as a result of separations or divorces. The majority of single parents are people at least 55 years and older, and 80% of them are single mothers (ISTAT, 2012). Parallel to the growth of single-parent households has been the growth of one-person households. Today they amount to almost one out of three families, increasing from 24.9% in 2001 to 31.2% in 2011 (ISTAT, 2013). Among this group 54.4% are aged 60 years and older, and once again women are the majorities in these families (Ministero del Lavoro e delle Politiche Sociali, 2013).

The trends noted above outline a progressive movement toward smaller and smaller family units, which often have women at their center—women who are often overburdened by providing care for both children and elderly parents as well as for themselves. In addition, this progressive atomization of the family also affects the web of parental and kin support. In general, familial solidarity is still strong in Italy, partially due to geographic proximity: 5.5% of families have a relative in the same building, 11.9% live less than a kilometer away, and 11.9% live in the same town (Glucksmann & Lyon, 2006; ISTAT, 2013a; Saraceno, 2003a). However, in recent years there has been a progressive restructuring of the informal web of support provided by relatives outside of the nuclear family (Zanatta, 2005). According to a study published in 2002, the percentage of families that has received support from this network has been declining from 23% in 1983 to 14% in 1998 (Sabbadini, 2002). Particularly significant for this study is the decline in support for families that have elders in their care: from 28.9% to 15.8% (Zanatta, 2005, p. 270).

The decreased ability to provide care, however, is not only due to demographic developments. Changes in women's participation in the labor market are also a factor. While women in Italy have entered the labor market later than in other European countries, their participation has been growing steadily for the last forty years both in full and part-time jobs. According to the OECD, in fact, the rate of labor market participation for women aged 15 to 64 has increased from 38.8% in 1981 to 55.2% in 2014 (OECD, 2015). And this trend is expected to increase for two reasons: on the one hand because European Union policies and directives are increasingly aiming at equalizing gender participation in the labor market and on the other because women will have to wait longer to retire (Naldini & DaRoit, 2010). The pension reform of 2012, following many others since the late 1990s, has delayed retirement age for both men and women, bringing it to 66 years of age. For men the change is immediate; for women it will happen gradually and become final in 2018 (INPS, 2013). This change is particularly important since the average age of women who care for elderly dependents is 61 years of age, so the upward shift in the retirement age greatly impacts their ability to provide care. These women are already under a lot of "care pressure," often providing simultaneous care for grandchildren and aging parents (Polverini et al., 2004; Rizza & Santangelo, 2014).

THE WELFARE STATE

The weakening of the familial structure, a pivotal element in the Italian welfare system, has not corresponded with a strengthening of the welfare state in providing services. Italy, historically, falls under a model of welfare state defined as the Mediterranean model (Da Roit & Sabatinelli, 2005; Naldini, 2003) or, alternatively, as a *familialist regime* (Esping-Andersen, 1999). This model is characterized by a low level of support for families with children, by limited public services for both children and the elderly, and by a shortage of policies that reconcile care and paid work (Bertani, 20013; Saraceno, 2003). In this care regime, family members have a legal obligation to care for dependent relatives, whereas public provisions for care are limited. Families' obligations for the financial and physical well-being of dependent family members go well beyond the nuclear family and also include parents, siblings, sons, and daughters-in-law. The state, on the other hand, does not assume any financial burden for the family/kinship-dependent members until all means of kin legally responsible for the elder dependent are thoroughly investigated (Naldini, 2003, p. 123). This is often a source of frustration for families. As one of my respondents explained in an interview:

> I tried to ask for some level of economic support for my mother but the social services told me that they could not intervene because my mother still had more than 3500 euros on her account... I tried to explain to them that this was the money she was saving for her own funeral but they said that there was nothing they could do. While she had that money in the bank they could not intervene.[4]

The strong reliance on families, a centerpiece of cultural and political development of the Italian welfare state, is also the main reason why family policies in Italy have remained underdeveloped (Naldini & Iurado, 2009; van Hooren, 2011). This underdevelopment is particularly glaring as far as policies for the elderly are concerned. According to sociologists Naldini and Saraceno (2008, p. 738), "Public policies at the national and local levels are largely inadequate as regards to meeting the needs of a growing population of frail elderly. Italy has, in fact, one of the lowest levels of coverage within the EU regarding services for the frail elderly." Italy, unlike many other aging countries in the world, has not undertaken a substantial national reform concerning eldercare policies. Overall social spending dedicated to long-term care continues to remain low (Da Roit, 2010) and it is likely to decrease even further due to current efforts aimed at reducing the national debt (Naletto, 2014).

The lack of national policies is hardly the only problem; access to public provisions and services is also impeded by the structural organization of the Italian welfare state. Since 1970s, the responsibility for social care and assistances has been progressively decentralized and increasingly assigned to regional and local authorities (Tediosi & Gabriele, 2010). This transformation, in turn, has generated a complicated system characterized by the presence of multiple actors that include the state, regions, municipalities, and local health agencies, who control and disburse different forms of funding often without internal coordination (Da Roit, 2010; Gori & Pelliccia, 2013; Spano, 2006, p. 20). The result is that even when services are available, families are often unaware of their existence and even when they are, the complexity of the procedures and the time-consuming tasks associated with requesting such services often deter families from obtaining them (personal interviews referenced in Chapter 6, Spano, 2006).

The low provision of welfare services is also connected to a widespread cultural model that values intergenerational support over other forms of long-term care. These deep-rooted cultural norms regarding the family and the elders, together with a perceived low quality of public institutions and high costs of private ones, often make families choose to incorporate the elders in their own family nucleus or, alternatively, to keep them in their own homes by providing extensive support. As a result of these factors, institutionalization rates in Italy have remained low. It is estimated that the actual institutionalization rate never surpassed 2% (with regional variation of 3% in the Northern regions and less than 1% in the Southern regions) and it is the lowest among European countries (Da Roit & Sabbatinelli, 2013). In addition to cultural norms, public discourse also enforces the importance of keeping elders out of institutions and in private homes. Recent legislation, such as law 328/2000 and the National Health Plan drafted by the Ministry for Health for 2006–2008, has reiterated the importance of maintaining elders at home within the family network (Ministero della Salute, 2006, p. 70) positing once again that the family should be at the center of social policies.

Low institutionalization rates of Italian elders is due not only to cultural norms but also to structural reasons; the limited availability of both private and public nursing or residential homes and their costs are also important limitations. A month at a *casa di riposo* (residential home care), usually restricted to the relatively self-sufficient elderly, may range from 1,400 euros, whereas the cost of a nursing home may be as high as 2,500 euros per month[5] (www.casariposo.org). According to a study conducted by the Osservatorio Terza Età/Aging Society, only 5% of the elders that make use of residential services receive total coverage from the state. For 62% costs of their stay fall upon themselves or their families; in 33% of the cases the costs are partially covered by the national healthcare system (Osservatorio Terza Età/Aging Society, 2006; Polverini et al., 2004).[6] Finally, admission to public residential institutions, which usually have lower costs, is not easy, and, at least in Piedmont (the region in which I conducted my research), involves a waiting list of at least 2 years (personal communication).

An option more often pursued by families who try to maintain their elders in their own homes is some form of state-provided homecare services. However, the state and local bodies such as regions and municipalities have not been able to coordinate a coherent provision and the supply is still insufficient (Barbabella, Chiatti, Di Rosa, & Gori 2013; DaRoit, 2007). Nevertheless, some forms of home care are provided by National Health System. For example, the *Assistenza Domiciliare Programmata* (Programmed Home Care Assistance) provides medical home care to patients who are unable to visit their general practitioner and the *Assistenza Domiciliare Integrata* (Integrated Home Care Assistance) is offered to terminal patients, patients affected by severe pathologies, patients who are temporarily disabled, or patients who have been prematurely discharged from the hospital (Polverini et al., 2004). These services, however, offer, at most, short daily visits and presuppose that most long-term care is done by family members or hired home eldercare assistants (personal experience). Other services that may be provided by different municipalities through a service called *Servizio di Assistenza Domiciliare* (Home Care Service) include help with housework, shopping, purchase of medicines, transport, companionship, and in case of extreme disability, personal services including hairdressing, manicures, and pedicures. Some municipalities also offer meal service to people 65 years old and over (Polverini et al., 2004). However, these services exist only in some geographic areas and do not reach more than 3% of the elderly population (Pesaresi & Gori, 2005). Furthermore, even when available, these services provide only a limited number of hours of support—some of the families interviewed for this project mentioned a maximum of 6 hours per week (personal interviews referenced in Chapter 6)—and they do not provide a viable alternative for either institutionalization or extended informal homecare (Da Roit, 2007, p. 252).

Although social care and services related to it are relatively underdeveloped in Italy, the tendency to monetize the provision of care is more common. Cash transfers began to become relatively common in Italy in the 1990s where they took different forms (Gori & Lamura, 2009; Gori & Torre, 2001) and, like services, they are administered by the state, regions, or municipalities. Among the different forms, perhaps the most common has been the *Indennita' di Accompagnamento* (State Attendance Allowance), a national allowance established in the 1980s and provided to citizens who either are unable to walk without assistance or need assistance in carrying out the basic activities of daily living (Polverini et al., 2004; van Hooren, 2011). This cash transfer, a national cash benefit scheme paid for by the National Social Security Institute (INPS), grants the highest monetary allowance to disabled civilians, providing a monthly stipend that in 2013 amounted to €499.27.[7] This benefit is not means-tested, but is conditional on certification of (severe) disability by the health authorities. The allowance is given directly to the disabled elder who may spend it at his or her own discretion with no strings attached (Da Roit, 2007; Gori & Torre, 2001).

Other forms of cash provisions granted by the state include the *Indennità Civile* (Civil Disability), which in case of a disability of 74% or more entitles the beneficiary to a means-tested monthly invalidity allowance, or, in case of total disability, to a disability pension. Other national measures include worker's disability allowance and a worker's disability pension provided by the National Institute for Social Security, as well as a few others (Polverini et al., 2004).

In the mid-1990s, keeping with similar trends of monetarization and marketization of care in other European countries, Italian local and regional authorities began to introduce new cash allowances—one being the *care allowance* (*assegno di cura*) geared to finance the care of dependent elders (Da Roit, 2007). These means-tested allowances offered by municipalities and local health agencies (Aziende Sanitarie Locali) may be in the form of cash or a tax credit and aim to support heavily dependent older people in disadvantaged economic conditions (Bettio & Verashchagina, 2010; Da Roit, 2007; Polverini et al., 2004). The allowances range between €387 and €1,291[8] depending on the level of disability and the means of the elder, however, and vary considerably among granting institutions. Nor are they evenly distributed across the country (Da Roit, 2007; Gori & Torri, 2001). Another common cash allowance is the *foster allowance* (*affidamento famigliare*), which involves a small reimbursement offered to families who care for an elder. This allowance ranges between €150 and €300[9] depending on the degree of disability of the elder.

Notwithstanding the uneven distribution, cash allowances have increased the availability of monetary resources for some elders and their families. This availability, coupled with a relatively generous pension system, provided elders and their families with the capacity to acquire private services, opening the door to a progressive marketization of care. In the 1990s the demand for paid care began to grow, but the limited amount of funding provided by the state, coupled with a low supply of private sector alternatives (Glucksmann & Lyon, 2006), confined the search for alternatives and families began to turn toward the informal labor market. It is at that time that the need for extended care at low cost began to coincide with the increasing presence of immigrant women and men confined to the informal labor market (Da Roit, 2007; Scrinzi, 2004, p. 109).

From the mid-1990s onward home eldercare assistance in Italy has grown in numbers; it has spread in the territory, and it has become rooted in Italian society. In some ways, however, it has also remained unchanged. This was true in 2011 when I went to Italy to do follow-up interviews, and it continues to be true today according to the data and the reports coming from researchers based in Italy (Ambrosini, 2015; Banchero, Brizioli, & Trabucchi, 2013; Costa, 2013; Pasquinelli & Rusmini, 2013). In fact, notwithstanding the fact that the occupation has been affected by the economic crisis of 2008–2009 and its aftermath, the austerity programs of recent years and the growing difficulties that families experience in paying for care, home eldercare assistance remains the most common solution for short-term and long-term eldercare provision. Im/migrant women continue to be at the core of it too, albeit alongside a growing but still relatively small presence of Italian workers (Censis-ISMU, 2013; Unipol-Censis, 2014; Pasquinelli & Rusmini, 2013). To this day, despite a growing need widely expressed both by elderly citizens and their families, the Italian welfare state has neither been able nor willing to implement a full-fledged national reform on the matter. National legislation has not been able to move the discussion to the next step in order to define the national need for eldercare support and how to implement an integration of all sources of financing related to eldercare. In addition, very few resources have been allocated at the national level to address the needs of the elderly population. Public spending for caring services increased by only 13% between 2004 and 2010 going from 1.05% of the total GDP to 1.18% (Costa, 2013). This is not to say that there have been no efforts to insert at least a skeletal framework in a highly unregulated labor market, but these efforts have been implemented only at the regional and local level remaining highly fragmented, and varying greatly across and within different geographic areas. In addition, due to limited funding, the incentive offered to employers to hire home eldercare assistants formally instead of informally or to hire regionally trained and certified ones instead of "unskilled" ones was too small to actually promote any kind of significant change (Pasquinelli & Rusmini, 2013).

IMMIGRATION IN ITALY AND THE INFORMAL LABOR MARKET

Starting in the 1970s, Italy began to change from a country of outmigration to a country of immigration. Previously, Italy had been a country characterized by migratory movements to the United States, France, Germany, Belgium, Luxembourg, and Switzerland (Campani, 2004; Gabaccia, 2000; Pugliese, 2002). However, after the 1973 oil crisis and the progressive implementation of stricter immigration policies by most European countries, this trend began to be reversed and by 1975 the Italian migratory balance became positive for the first time, with the number of immigrants noticeably higher than that of emigrants (Castles; 2000; Colombo & Sciortino; 2004; Schierup et al., 2006, p. 163). By the early 1980s, Northern Italy had already become an important destination for migratory fluxes with considerable numbers entering every year (Pugliese, 2002). However, it was in the 1990s, with the collapse of the Soviet Union and the imposition of neoliberal economic policies across the world, that the numbers of im/migrant workers began to grow quickly. From around 300,000 at the beginning of the 1980s (Schierup et al., 2006, p. 164), the immigrant population grew to almost 2 million in 2004 and reached 4.4 million at the beginning of 2013 (ISTAT, 2014); it now represents 7.4% of the total population residing in the country. The great majority of resident immigrants are concentrated in Northern and Central Italy. At the regional level, Lombardia, Emilia Romagna, Veneto, Lazio, and Piemonte have the highest number of foreigners, while the cities with the highest concentrations are Rome, Milan, and Turin with 252,582, 194,991, and 177,533, respectively (DEMO ISTAT, 2013; ISTAT, 2014 Noi Italia). Women account for more than half of this population—reaching 53% in 2013 (Caritas, 2013)—and they are the majority in a great number of communities including the: Romanian, Ukrainian, Filipino, Moldovan, Peruvian, Ecuadorian and Sri Lankan—as Table 3.2 demonstrates—which confirms patterns of feminization in migration processes. Interestingly, the communities in which women are the majority are also the ones with a greater participation in home eldercare assistance.

Together with the regular resident population, Italy has been hosting a large population of irregular immigrants. Among the reasons Italy was attractive were a relatively lax border control, and a fair availability of irregular, flexible, low-end jobs open to irregular im/migrants[10] (Schierup, 2006, p. 187). The migratory phenomenon in Italy has to be understood in the context of a large informal economy in which irregular employment is very common and can absorb the great majority of migrants (Anthias & Lazarides, 2000). Throughout the 1980s Italy underwent a profound economic transformation away from heavy manufacturing, which was largely concentrated in the hands of a few giant factories such as Fiat or Parmalat, toward the development of a large secondary sector of small and medium-sized businesses, often family run (Ambrosini, 2001; Calavita, 2005, pp. 54–56). Scattered over the territory, these deceptively modest businesses have created niches within national and international markets, concentrating on just-in-time production, and reducing the cost of labor (Calavita, 2005). Many of these businesses are part of the vast underground economy, and

Table 3.2. Largest Migrant Communities Present in Italy According to Nationality and Gender on January 1, 2001

Nationality	Females	Males	Total
Romania	529,265	439,311	968, 576
Albania	223,275	259,352	482,627
Morocco	197,518	254,906	452,424
China	101,516	108,418	209,934
Ukraine	160,113	40,617	200,730
Philippines	77,595	56,559	134,154
Moldova	87,951	42,997	130,948
India	47,590	73,446	121,036
Poland	77,603	31,415	109,018
Tunisia	38,856	67,435	106,291
Peru	39,310	59,293	98,603
Ecuador	37,985	53,640	91,625
Egypt	27,525	62,840	90,365
Macedonia	39,570	50,330	89,900
Bangladesh	26,809	55,642	82,451
Sri Lanka	36,087	45,007	81,094

Source: ISTAT (2011).

although they employ a regular workforce, they often supplement it with off the books employment (Calavita, 2005, p. 55). In other words, these businesses helped to create a primary and secondary labor market, with the secondary market offering only unstable, undesirable jobs with no security and uncertain prospects. The widespread practices of these businesses have led to the rise in demand for a cheap, flexible, nondemanding labor force, one often composed of young people living with their families, migrants, and frequently women (Anthias & Lazarides, 2000). Alongside the increased need for a flexible workforce in light manufacturing, construction, and agriculture, Italy began to experience an increased need for domestic and carework, which, to this day, remains one of the most important areas of immigrant participation in the labor market (Reyneri, 2011).

In addition to transformations in the labor market, what made Italy attractive to foreign im/migrants was the fact that, together with Spain and Greece, it was considered a backdoor to the rest of Europe (Calavita, 2005). After the oil crisis of 1973–1984, countries that had been attracting im/migrants for a long time such as France, England, and Germany began to close their doors to noncitizens. It was then that im/migrants began to look at Italy as a possible point of entry. Until the early 1990s, border controls in Italy were not as strict as those of Northern European countries and its geographic configuration made it possible to reach it by water, making it particularly attractive for im/migrants coming from Northern Africa and Eastern Europe (Chell-Robinson, 2000; Faedda, 2014). Furthermore, because of the many bilateral immigration agreements that Italy has entered over the years, it was a country still easily accessible through tourist visas (Schierup et al., 2006), which, according to Frontex (the European Agency for the Management of Operational Cooperation at the External Borders of the Member States of the European Union), continues to be the most common mode of entry for potential irregular immigrants (2013).

Finally, another factor that explained the growing influx of migrants to the country was and still is its uncertain immigration policies. Until 1986, Italy lacked comprehensive legislation concerning immigration and to this day it maintains an ambivalent position on the issue—on the one hand joining the rest of Europe and the United States in attempting to close its borders, and on the other hand periodically providing amnesties for irregular immigrants already present in the country.

Table 3.3 shows that, from 1998 onward, legislation concerning migration became progressively more restrictive, following the pattern already established in other countries of the Global North. However, every tightening of the screw was followed by amnesty for irregular workers already present in the country. This apparently contradictory behavior reflects two trends that have developed in the past 20 years: on the one hand media and politicians have developed a language, practices and policies that depict, treat and present immigration as a crisis and/or an emergency that requires extremes measures, on the other hand, the labor market has quietly absorbed many of these im/migrants taking advantage of the new possibilities that these workers represent (Ambrosini, 2013). Although apparently antithetical, these two processes are actually functional to one another. Italy, particularly after 2001, began to follow other wealthy, postindustrial countries in the attempt to "securitize" its borders in order to keep "unwanted others" out (Castles, De Haan, & Miller, 2013). To achieve these goals the Italian Parliament drafted increasingly more restrictive immigration laws, described in detail in Table 3.3, which culminated with the Law n.189, also known as the Bossi/Fini,[11] and this was further bolstered by the Security Package of 2008, which declared irregular immigration a crime—a decision reversed only in 2014 due to claims of unconstitutionality raised by the European Union.

Acknowledging the important role of im/migrant labor not only in providing a cheap and flexible workforce, but also in providing a solution to the growing need for care, the welfare state increasingly tied regularization processes and legality to labor. The state did so in many ways: by creating and enhancing a system of quotas tied to specific needs in the labor market, by providing amnesties for irregular migrants already residing in the countries[12] and working in specific sectors of the labor market, and by pushing the onus of regularization onto employers. By alternatively rejecting and regularizing immigrants, the state sends contradictory messages to both immigrants and civil society at

Table 3.3. Review of Immigration Law from 1986 to 2012

Law	Description
Law n 943, 30/12 1986 Renewed through Act n.81, 1988	This law, the first Italian law on immigration, proposed an amnesty for the irregular migrants residing in the country, and laid down provisions for subsequent immigration. It introduced parity of treatment between foreign and Italian workers concerning access to social benefits and welfare services. It ensured migrants' rights to family reunion, and included employers' sanctions in case of smuggling or exploitation. It also introduced the opportunity to enter the country through the direct call of an Italian employer. The first regularization, which encompassed 105,000 migrant workers, required migrants to be irregularly employed by an employer willing to "regularize" them, but applications of job seekers were also accepted.
Law n.39, 28/02 1990 (from a decree of 30/12 1989) known as the "Martelli Law"	The new law confirmed the equality of rights between foreigners and Italians, tightened the conditions for entry into the country, but at the same time enlarged the margins for the regularization of those already present in the country. The law sealed the border except for very small, programmed flows or annual quotas of workers. The amnesty promoted through this law required migrants to prove that they had been living in Italy before the end of 1989. It allowed for the regularization of 218,000 workers.
The New Nationality Law, Act n.91 5/2 1992	The law raised the period required to obtain citizenship from 5 to 10 years, but reduced the period to 4 years for EU citizens, and to 3 years for people of Italian origin.
Decree-Law 489/95 also known as the "Dini Decree" (renewed as DL 376/96)	The decree provided more restrictive terms concerning the borders and the expulsion of illegal immigrants, but at the same time allowed for a new amnesty for all the migrants already working in the country. The amnesty, which had stricter requirements compared to the previous one (a job offer by an employer was needed to apply) affected 248,000 people.
Law n.40, 06/3 1998 also known as the "Turco-Napolitano Law"	This is considered the most ambitious attempt to reorganize immigration policies in Italy and seriously addresses the issue of long-term incorporation of migrants in society and in the welfare system. The law had three main objectives: a restructuring of workers' fluxes in the country, the effective prevention of irregular immigration, and the integration of migrants already residing in the country. The law established that annual quotas would be determined by the President of the Council of Ministers and the Parliament according to the needs of the labor market. The law also clarified the additional conditions based on which migrants could enter and reside legally in the country: through national seasonal quotas, a work contract with an Italian employer, and the sponsorship of an Italian resident. Residence permits would be issued for 2 years and renewed if conditions (usually formal employment) continued to be met. Workers who had lost their jobs were given a year to find new employment. Moreover, after 5 years of continued legal status the residence permit would give way to a Residence Card (*Carta di Soggiorno*), open-ended in duration. It also expanded the rights of foreigners within Italy: the right to equal treatment in the workplace, access to the universal healthcare system, and for the irregular, the right to urgent care and the right to attend public school. At the same time, the irregular status of the workers began to be equated with illegality and the law foresaw the possibility of detaining illegal immigrants in special centers of residence and assistance. The amnesty connected to this law had the same requirements as the one in 1996 and it allowed for the regularization of 217,000 workers.

(continued)

Table 3.3. Continued

Law n.189, 30/7 2002 also known as the "Bossi-Fini Law"	This law's main concern was to demonstrate "below-zero tolerance" for illegal immigration and to tighten the connection between work and legal status. According to this law, each year the Prime Minister will decide the quota of workers that could be admitted for the following year, with no limitations for high-skilled workers. Other non-EU immigrants will be allowed entry in Italy only if in possession of a Residence Contract (*Contratto di Soggiorno*), a contract of dependent employment signed by an employer and the migrant worker. The contract must provide for accommodation and the payment of travel expenses for the workers to return to their country of origin. When the contract expires the worker must return to the country of origin. (The law eliminated the sponsor system.) Family reunification is allowed only for migrants with a regular residence permit and is limited only to *first-degree* relatives. Residence permits are issued for a maximum of 2 years, and renewals must be requested 3 months before expiration even if the worker has an open-ended contract. If at the time of renewal the worker does not have a job she or he will be offered a 6-month grace time to find another job, after which no further renewal will be granted. The Residence Card (*Carta di Soggiorno*) can still be obtained, but only after 6 years of continued legal residence and not 5 years. All non-EU citizens requesting a Residence Permit (*Permesso di Soggiorno*) have to be fingerprinted. Irregular immigrants will be deported, with suspected illegal immigrants detained in specific centers controlled by the police. Again the law includes a provision to regularize irregular workers, with specific attention to domestic and care workers. This time it is an employer-driven regularization, meaning that employers have to request it, pay for it, and provide documentation. The 2002 law allowed for the regularization of a total of 634,728 illegal immigrants (more than all the previous amnesties together).
Security Law 94/July 2009	Illegal immigration becomes **a crime**, thus all public officers and public workers must report the presence of an illegal immigrant. Illegal immigrants are liable to pay a fine and can now be detained by the authorities for more than 6 months. Each petition made to the **public administration**, such as requests for money transfers, much be accompanied by the applicant's permanent residency permit, with the exception of applications for healthcare, school, and birth certificates. **Helping an illegal immigrant come to Italy**, or housing irregular migrants, is now prosecutable as a crime (up to 3 years in prison). Italian teachers must report irregular children. Legal immigrants **married** to an Italian must wait 2 years to obtain Italian citizenship. The law allows for the formation of **unarmed citizen patrol groups**. Connected to the passage of the security law there is a corresponding amnesty that allows for the regularization of 294,000 foreign workers.
September 2012	Prime Minister Monti allows for a new regularization of irregular workers regularly employed in Italian homes and enterprises. Immigrant workers need to have been employed for a minimum of 3 months. The regularization process this time involves 130,000 requests.
April 2014	The lower house of the Italian Parliament agreed with the Senate to abolish the crime of entering or staying in the country without a permit. Irregular immigrants will still be deported, but they will not be held in prison for the "crime" of migrating.

Source: Elaboration of the author from material provided by Ambrosini (2015), Barbagli, Colombo, and Sciortino (2004), Calavita (2005), Chell (2000), Merrill (2006), Schierup et al. (2006), and Triandafyllidou and Marchetti (2014).

large. On the one hand the state *normalizes* irregular migration by making it an inevitable rite of passage in the life of immigrants to Italy; on the other hand it provides civil society, politicians, and the media with the tools to keep immigrants constantly balancing on a fine line between acceptance and tolerance, between being needed and being rejected. This constant ambiguity helps to keep immigrant workers in precarious and vulnerable positions, which, in turn, pushes them into very specific sectors of the labor market in which precariousness and vulnerability are the daily bread. Unlike native workers who need to be socialized into the contemporary dogmas of flexibility and precariousness, im/migrant workers are, due to these processes, structurally located in them. In addition, these processes are also gendered because they tend to privilege women over men, albeit in an indirect way as we will see in the next section.

LEGISLATION REGARDING DOMESTIC AND CARE WORK

The connection between migration and domestic work in Italy started very early. Beginning in the mid-1960s, women from Eritrea, the Philippines, Cape Verde Islands, Salvador, Somalia, and Sri Lanka began to enter the country, often with the mediation of the Catholic Church, to come to work in private homes as domestic workers (Campani, 2007).[13] Prior to 1986, domestic work was the only channel available to im/migrant workers that enabled them to enter Italy with a work permit (Reyneri, 2001). In these years control of overseas workers occurred through government circulars issued by the Ministry of Labor and Social Welfare and the Foreign Ministry (Andall, 2000). To enter the country, a prospective im/migrant domestic worker had to present, together with a certification of good health and some proof of moral and civic integrity, a request to the diplomatic or consular bodies of their own countries.

> These applications would then be sent by these bodies to the Department for the Placement of Workers (*Direzione Generale del Collocamento della Manodopera*), which, in turn, allocated workers to the provincial offices (*Ufficio provinciale del Lavoro*) according to their estimated need. The provincial offices would then contact prospective employers with a choice of workers (Andall, 2000, pp. 122–123).

This system lasted until 1986 when the government passed a more comprehensive law on immigration. Nevertheless, domestic work continued to offer a privileged channel of entry even after that year. In the 1990s, the yearly inflow of domestic workers continued to be significantly higher than that of other im/migrant workers: 10,000–12,000 a year versus 3,000–4,000 per year. Between 1965 and 1990, the number of female immigrants increased by 63%, whereas the male number increased by 58% (Campani, 2007).

These patterns continued at least until 1995 when domestic work began to be regulated by national labor demand control and new entries decreased dramatically (Reyneri, 2001). The need for domestic and care work, however, did not decrease and the yearly quotas for the entry of domestic workers were not sufficient to satisfy the increased demand. It was at this time that most of this demand began to be filled by irregular female im/migrants coming from different areas of the world, ranging from Eastern Europe to sub-Saharan Africa and from Southeast Asia to South America. The full scope of the presence of im/migrant workers in the domestic and care labor market, however, did not emerge until July 2002 when the Italian center-right government, led by Prime Minister Silvio Berlusconi, presented the Bossi-Fini law. As mentioned before, the law, while enforcing more restrictive rules regarding immigration overall, also included an amnesty that acknowledged the role of im/migrant labor in fulfilling the need for domestic work and eldercare. Article 33 of this law, in fact, allowed for the regularization of all irregular immigrants currently working in private families either as domestic or home eldercare[14] assistants.

The amnesty, which in September 2002 was followed by a more inclusive one involving all dependent workers in subordinate employment,[15] allowed for the regularization of a total of 634,728 irregular immigrants (Ministero dell'Interno, 2004). Of the total requests for regularization, 52% concerned dependent workers in different sectors, whereas the other half, 341,121 requests, concerned domestic workers and home eldercare assistants, respectively 27.6% and 20.4% (ISMU, 2005). This first regularization was followed by less successful ones in 2009 with 300,000 requests and in 2012 with circa 135,000 requests, where, once again, the largest numbers were those of domestic and eldercare workers. Though some of the requests for regularization as domestic and home eldercare assistants may have been a scheme to obtain a regular residence permit (Sarti, 2004), the total number of requests in the domestic and care sector revealed a great need for these positions in the Italian labor market—a need that remains unquantifiable because, as some authors have pointed out, regularizations do not "catch" all irregular workers (see among others Zucchetti, 2004).

Regularizations of domestic and care workers did not happen only at the national level; regional agreements on immigration also affected the labor market. As sociologist Maurizio Ambrosini (2013, p. 15) pointed out, the 2004 and 2007 enlargements of the European Union have also allowed for the regularization of thousands of immigrants previously considered irregular. Among the many that gained regular status were immigrants from Cyprus, the Czech Republic, Estonia, Hungary, Latvia, Lithuania, Malta, Poland, Slovakia, and Slovenia first, followed later on by those from Romania and Bulgaria. Changes of the political order at the regional level allowed these workers not only to go from irregular to regular status but also to gain a great deal of mobility, allowing many to engage in a short-term circulatory migration instead of a long-term one, and in many cases facilitating the choice of informal employment.

Different immigration policies both at the regional and the local level helped generate a highly segmented labor force ranging from privileged migrants who can easily return to their countries for extended periods of times and who may be interested in both live-in positions or short-term jobs, to regular immigrants who can negotiate more freely with their employers because of their position vis-à-vis immigration laws, to irregular im/migrants who are instead extremely vulnerable because of their position with respect to the law but also because of the widespread negative campaign against them.

CONCLUSIONS

This chapter explored how global and regional macroprocesses become embedded in the local reality of one specific country, in this case Italy, generating new realities and new processes. Specifically, it looked at how the feminization of migration generated through political and economic transformations both in sending and receiving countries came to intersect with the growing need for short-term and long-term eldercare in Italy, transforming the Italian care regime from a family-based one to a "migrant in the family" one as suggested by Bettio, Simonazzi, and Villa (2006, p. 272).

To this day the exact number of domestic and care workers operating in Italy remains unknown due to the fact that many of these labor relations happen in the gray area of informal labor. Nevertheless, it is estimated that this occupation currently involves between 500,000 and 1,600,000 workers (Ambrosini, 2015; Censis-Fondazione ISMU, 2013). In addition, it is uncontroversial that the need for this type of labor has been growing steadily, particularly since the 1990s, and the presence of im/migrant workers in this sector is by now considered vital and irreplaceable by both the Italian state and Italian families (Bonizzoni, 2013, p. 135; Catanzaro & Colombo, 2009; Sgritta, 2009). The Italian state is complicit in this arrangement in two ways: first, by choosing to pursue a politic of long-term care that instead of offering in-kind services, focuses almost exclusively on cash allowances without strings attached. By providing allowances and not services the welfare state inevitably pushes families toward looking for care in the market—a market that for many years did not involve options other than immigrant labor. Second, by choosing to adopt complex and often contradictory migration policies, the state directly and indirectly helps to manage and shape different migratory flows channeling im/migrant workers in a widely segmented labor market. The combination of restrictive policies on the one hand and regularizations at both the national and the regional level on the other have resulted, over time, in a landscape in which im/migrants experience a great deal of variation in terms of legal status, cross-border mobility, and migratory projects. These differences, in turn, work to produce a segmented labor force willing to accept extremely different wages, working conditions, and living arrangements. This is not a new phenomenon per se—Piore in 1979 already showed how new waves of migration tend to put pressure on the pay and working conditions of already-settled foreign workers; however, the phenomenon is intensified in this specific labor market due to the increased variation in immigrant status. Different statuses also provide access to different migratory journeys. Immigrants who have the ability to pursue pendulum migration ask employers for very different wages and working conditions than immigrants who are trying to settle in the country. This diversification of the market, in turn, provides Italian families with an extremely competitive and variegated market capable of responding to most needs at all wage levels while at the same time providing the welfare state with a quick and inexpensive fix for a complex issue.

NOTES

1 The term familialist was attributed to the Italian welfare state by Esping Andersen to define a welfare state that relies mostly on families for the provision of services.
2 The aging index is calculated as the number of persons 60 years old or over per hundred persons under age 15 years.
3 Well below the rate that would guarantee balance between births and deaths in the overall population, a rate set at 2.1 per woman.
4 Approximately US $3950.
5 Corresponding to approximately US $1,577 and $2,816.
6 According to the website of the Region Piemonte, expenses concerning the residential structures are distributed as follows: the room and board expenses are paid by the elders or their families, whereas the medical expenses are paid by the National Health Care System. If the income of the elders and their families is below a certain amount (including not only yearly income but also personal property) the municipality will provide some financial support. http://www.provincia.torino.it/sportellosociale/anziani/sa11
7 Approximately US $562 per month.
8 Between US $169 and $338.
9 Between US $203 and $406.
10 In the book I use the term im/migrant instead of either immigrant or migrants to emphasize that contemporary immigration involves both people with long-term migratory projects who plan to integrate in destination countries and people who do not plan to settle in or go back and forth between sending and receiving countries.
11 From the name of the politicians who promoted it.
12 Regularizations were offered in 1982, 1986, 1990, 1995, 1998, 2002, 2009, and 2012.

13 These women were, for the most part, at the forefront of the feminization of migration because they were among the first to migrate alone as primary migrants.

14 This is the time when the term "badante" becomes common in the Italian language and it becomes official through the Bossi-Fini law. Throughout the book I use the term home eldercare assistant instead of *badante* because, as do many other scholars, I consider the term "minders" offensive to both the workers and the elders for whom they care. Technically, the appropriate translation should be *homecare assistants* to also include all the workers who provide care to disabled people, but I chose to use *home eldercare assistants* to stress that the majority of these positions involve caring for the elders.

15 Decree-Law n.195 9/9/2002.

4

THE BURDEN OF LONG-TERM CARE

ITS CULTURAL, ECONOMIC, AND SOCIAL ASPECTS

> I wouldn't call what I need long-term care because my mother is terminally ill and her journey will not be much longer, but I do need help caring for her exactly like the women I have been interviewing need help caring for their elders. She now needs constant assistance, day and night. The ASL (Local Health Agency) has provided us with a nurse who comes every few days for 15–20 minutes but it is clear that the nurse expects somebody to provide the daily care and, honestly, some of the tasks are a bit daunting. The nurse has been training Annaliza and me to give her medications, to start and stop the infusions, but soon the two of us will not be enough to provide her with the comfort she needs. I work during the day and I have a family including an 18-month-old daughter. Annaliza [who used to do domestic work for my mother once a week] is now here all day, 5 days a week, sometimes 6 days. During the day she watches both my mother and my daughter and I do what I can in between interviews and research . . . then in the weekend we alternate with my aunts, but now we need somebody to provide care at night as well. The infusions need to be changed and my mother is in pain all the time and does not sleep but she does not want to go to the hospital and who would blame her . . . after the last experience at the emergency room (ER) it is clear that they do not have much patience for terminal patients . . . I honestly do not know how to handle all of this, it is eating me alive (personal journal entry February 22, 2004).

As seen in the previous chapters a combination of demographic, cultural, political, and economic factors has in the past 20 years placed increasing pressure on Italian families to provide care for their elders. This pressure, however, is not equally distributed among family members; rather it continues to fall for the most part on women, because the provision of care continues to be a "women's affair" (Alemani, 2004; Francavilla, Giannelli, Grotkowska, & Mieczyslaw, 2011; Piazza, 1997). These findings resonate with findings in many other parts of the global North where large numbers of women are struggling to find a balance between work and family, between domestic work and child care, and, increasingly, with care for elderly parents. The growing tendency of outsourcing domestic and care labor to immigrant women has been extensively explored in both the literature on: globalization, the feminization of migration and the global care chain (among them Anderson, 2000, Chang, 2000, Constable, 1997; Gamburd, 2000; Gutierrez-Rodriguez, 2010; Hochschild, 2000; Hondagneu-Sotelo, 2001; Lan, 2006; Lutz, 2008; Parreñas, 2001; Yeates, 2009). In much of that literature the argument that is often made is that the work that immigrant women perform as domestic workers and nannies allows women of the global North not only to lighten their load of reproductive work but it also allows them to pursue more satisfying careers, to achieve higher social status (Anderson, 2000; Yeates, 2009), and/or to dedicate themselves to more rewarding activities such as their children's education and extracurricular activities or philanthropic work. In addition, scholars and policy makers often tend to depict the choice of hiring immigrant labor simply as a desire to obtain cheap and flexible labor (Bettio, Simonazzi, & Villa, 2006; Ranci, 2001; Spano, 2006). To better understand this issue in this chapter I explore, through the words of family caregivers, what causes Italian family providers of long-term care to become employers of informal caregivers, how they negotiate an experience that for many is a new one, and how they select a prospective employee.

THE CAREGIVERS

The interviews I conducted during my research in Italy confirmed that the provision of care to disabled elders continues to be provided predominantly by women (Pickard, 2011). In 22 out of 28 cases, the main care providers were women. In only four cases were men the main providers, whereas in another two cases the care was shared by a mother and son. Most of the family caregivers were women in their early fifties to mid-sixties (a few were older), and they were working full time or had recently retired. In most cases, their families still relied on them for daily subsistence. They belonged to all strata of Italian society, ranging from the very affluent to the lower middle class. Most had tried, before becoming employers, to manage the situation by themselves. Certainly there were exceptions and there were a number of families who, from the beginning, chose to completely defer the care of their elders to either institutions or immigrant home eldercare assistants. However, the majority of the employers I encountered were caregivers who, after having tried to deal with the situation on their own for 1, 5, or 7 years decided to get help. Vanna, who took care of her 89-year-old mother, when asked about her experience with long-term care, provided the following description:

> My mother is affected by Parkinson's, senile dementia, and diabetes, I don't know what else she could have. She is 89 years old and she is completely out of her mind. She began to show signs of instability fifteen years ago and since then. . . . You can imagine, I can't take it any longer, I really can't. Today she was acting crazy because she wanted to eat sugar. She can't because she has diabetes, but she was so out of control that after hours of begging and pleading I gave her some. I don't care anymore. Do you know what it means to be exasperated?

Vanna's experience is not an isolated one. Rather it reflects the experience of most family caregivers who embark on the aging voyage of their loved ones. The quote summarizes how family caregivers struggle to keep up with a process that happens at different speeds but that, instead of getting better and becoming lighter over time, as in the case of child care, becomes more difficult to manage and deeply affects familial relationships.

HOW IT STARTS. . .

The first element that emerges from the interviews is that the amount of care needed by the elders is not fixed but changes over time. When it begins, usually all that is required is some supervision of daily activities, such as keeping an eye on a forgetful elder, buying groceries, paying bills, and/or taking care of occasional complex or heavy tasks. Cosimo, who provided assistance to his father-in-law, recollected:

> The current situation started last August after my father-in-law broke his femur. Since then he has become vulnerable and needs assistance. He is still independent, for the most part . . . he can take care of himself in terms of personal hygiene and can, if he feels like it, cook for himself, but he no longer feels confident.

For some fortunate ones, the needs of the frail elder had remained at this level—support and company for a few hours a day. For the majority, however, the need for care had increased over time, either from the slow progression into a form of dementia, the faster onset of a disease, or the result of a surgery. In all such cases the amount of care required for the elders increased first to full working days and then to 24 hours a day, 7 days a week. Claudia, who for 5 years had taken care of both of her parents, explained her situation:

> My odyssey began five years ago when my mother had surgery to replace her knee. Up to that moment, my parents were completely independent and needed only a house cleaner once in a while to help them with the most demanding tasks. I used to work back then and I didn't have much time for them. After the surgery, however, my mom became more and more insecure. . . . So I decided to leave my job to help them out. Progressively my mother's condition got worse. She began to have ischemic episodes that first left her in a wheel chair, and then killed her last December. My father, who is now 94 years old, is the only one left and he too needs full-time assistance.

Claudia's experience was by no means uncommon among the respondents. Many families with perfectly functioning elderly family members found themselves, over the years, becoming engulfed in a growing need for long-term care that, in an absence of publicly provided services or other feasible alternatives, made it very difficult to maintain a balance between care and work. In a few cases, this heightened need for care even forced family caregivers to leave their jobs to dedicate themselves full time to managing the elders' physical and mental decline. Furthermore, these situations, even if often seemingly dire and difficult to manage, were not necessarily short-term problems, and families often ended up being caught in them for years. Benedetta, who provided assistance for her 80-year-old mother, explained:

> We have been in this situation for ten years. . . . When we first brought my mother to the doctor they gave her six months to live. That happened ten years ago but she is still among us. It is a very difficult situation because my mother suffers from Alzheimer's, Parkinson's and diabetes, and she needs full-time assistance. Everybody commends us for what we have done for her.

The situation can be further complicated when parents on both sides of the family need extended care. Orazio, whose mother was affected by senile dementia, described it as follows:

> I finally thought that I had a handle on the situation when I hired a home eldercare assistant to take care of my mother . . . although the situation is once again degenerating, because my mom is now beginning to suffer nocturnal incontinence and she doesn't want to wear diapers. Up to this moment, the person who works for her has been getting up to help her,

> but I cannot ask her to do it forever. I will have to hire somebody else for the night. And now, on top of all this, my mother-in-law's health has begun to decline--she has lost the use of her legs. We are waiting for a hip replacement but in the meantime . . . we had to hire somebody for her too.

THE GENDERED DIMENSION OF LONG-TERM CARE

Such intensive need for care and assistance places a huge load on families in terms of both emotional and physical commitment. Women, in particular, continue to be the ones who end up with the greatest burden. It is important to mention that although there were six men among the care providers interviewed, women were still considered the main providers of care in all the families. Where brothers and sisters were present, it was often the sisters who took on the full load of care. Martina, who assisted both her elderly parents, explained the family dynamics:

> We are three sisters and one brother. I do most of the care, but my sisters in one way or another support me. My brother, instead, is absolutely uninterested. He comes once a month, like the doctor. He has no interest in them, not even a phone call for my mother whose mind still works fine. Nothing.

Even when the brothers played a fuller part, at least in terms of economic and managerial support, most women felt that they were better equipped to provide care, which reflects the traditional gendered division of labor. Claudia, unlike her brother, lives next door to her father. She recounts:

> My brother offers me all the support I need. He helps with the economic aspect of care, which is not a small matter, but also in helping me make decisions and when there are important things to do, like taking [my father] to the doctor, or to obtain the disability certificate. . . . He helps me, but I'm the one that solves my father's problems on a daily basis . . . maybe because a woman is more inclined to do these sorts of things.

Independent of family circumstances, the women who cared for elderly relatives full time were often caught between two care demands: for the elder and for their own families. Martina, who cared for both of her parents, lucidly described the tensions:

> [To care for my parents] I had to give up [looking after] myself and my needs, and even those of my husband. On top I often feel split. . . . I'm

> confused, especially when I'm really tired, about what I have done for them or for us. Did I buy the milk for them or for us? I can't always remember what I have done in my house and what I have done in my parents' house, because naturally I have to split myself between the places—my husband complains that I think only about them and not us.

The mention of a husband upset by the limitations placed on the family lifestyle by the extensive amount of care provided to the older person was a common thread across the interviews, an added element of stress to the already overextended lives of most of the women. However, it was not only husbands who complained. As Orazio remarked, "[My mother's situation] adds difficulties to my relationship with my wife. I mean, my wife is very understanding and available, but she thinks that there should be a limit to the time I spend with my mother. She thinks that my mother had her life and we need to have one too." Many families that care for one or more disabled elders lose the ability to live an autonomous life. Among the participants, even when the help of a home eldercare assistant was available, most needed "to fill in" on the weekend or during holidays, and vacations were no longer considered feasible. This loss of control over one's life was considered particularly galling because it came at a time when most of the families had finished raising their own children and many had retired; they were planning to rest and to have a more carefree lifestyle. Vilma elaborated:

> To have a parent so dependent, so needy [it] changes your life. It is a traumatic event, because I have grown children and my husband and I have gotten used to coming and going whenever we wanted, to make plans, to leave on the spur of the moment; and now all that freedom is taken away. . . . It is a fine line and especially for a woman it is difficult to maintain a balance.

The necessity of living two lives, one for themselves and one for the elders in their care, not only took a great physical and emotional toll on care providers but also on their well-being. Many of the women interviewed mentioned that they had developed stress-related ailments that affected them both physically and mentally. The difficulties involved in caring for elderly parents or relatives were amplified because many of the elders, due to their ailments and their physical and mental decline, were often in a bad mood, difficult to deal with, or outright nonsensical. Gaia, whose mother was 94 years of age, described such difficulties well:

> I don't want to exaggerate, but I think that because of my mom's situation I had entered a state of depression. Every time she sees me, it is a fight. As soon as I walk into the house she accuses me: "You changed my overcoat,

you took my umbrella, you switched my scissors, you took all the things that were in the dining room's cabinets." And I try to explain, to tell her that is not true, but every time she attacks me and I end up responding and screaming.

The moodiness of the elders, the bouts of senile dementia, and the anger that often emerges from difficulties related to a body or a mind that increasingly fails them are common problems described by all the caregivers and the closer the caregiver is to the elders the stronger the problem. Most caregivers, in fact, even though understanding that these behaviors are linked to the aging process are not able to see them simply as such. For many the interactions with the elders are extremely difficult because they continue to see them first and foremost as husbands/wives, fathers/mothers, or aunts/uncles, and only secondarily as elderly people. Fiore, a 77-year-old woman who cares for her 92-year-old husband explained:

> In recent months he has begun to accuse me of infidelities, he calls me names, he tells me stories that he makes up in his head . . . I talked to his doctor and he explained that it is common among people who are affected by senile dementia . . . they make up these movies in their head and they become real. I know what it is, I understand it, but at the same time I cannot forgive him. I cook for him, clean after him but I no longer speak to him. I can't forgive him. . . .

These tensions end up deeply affecting lifelong relationships among family members and in the end also affect the quality of the care provided to the elders. It is a running thread through the quotes that the transformation of the elders into irrational and capricious beings, even when intellectually understood, remained an emotionally difficult adjustment for family caregivers to make.

In addition to the emotional and physical toll of caring for the elders, another aspect that deeply concerned many Italian families was the cost of extended care. Among the participants, only two of the more affluent family members did not mention costs, but all the others talked about the economic difficulties associated with the provision of good care. Belinda explained her household's situation:

> My father lives with us and has a monthly pension of 540 euros.[1] You wouldn't believe it but with that money I can barely pay for everything he needs. . . . First he needs medications . . . and now that he has this esophagus problem he eats only baby food, which is very expensive. . . . Now out of desperation, I hired this Peruvian lady who comes for two hours every evening while I'm [working] at the diner, but he is still alone from 8 pm to midnight when I come home from work, I can't pay for all that. . . . I give him a sleeping pill and hope for the best.

According to all the interviewees, the pensions of the older family members were not sufficient to cover all the care expenses, so many family caregivers had to contribute financially to ensure proper care. The costs attached to eldercare, particularly when distant relatives were concerned, were often expenses that the family had not budgeted for, which caused great difficulties both in terms of providing the necessary time for care and maintaining its quality.

ELDERS AND RESIDENTIAL FACILITIES

In spite of the complex emotions and the practical difficulties in providing full-time care for elderly parents and relatives, 24 of the 28 families were resistant to the idea of placing them in residential homes. Many considered the option a form of abandonment and betrayal, and for these reasons residential facilities were generally seen as the solution of last resort. Vilma elaborated on these thoughts:

> I wouldn't [put her in a residential facility] because I know she wouldn't want me to. It would be going against her will, even if I think that the facilities of today are no longer what they used to be, because now they have specialized personnel. . . . . I think that if you have offspring, if you have somebody that, in a way or another, can care for you [that is how it should be].

For others the notion of keeping the dependent older person at home was not even discussed: it was regarded as a cultural norm, as "what people do." Alberto, who shared his house with his 79-year-old father, whom his wife cared for, explained how the arrangement came about:

> My father asked to live with us, but he didn't need to. It was implied that he should live with us. He expected it, maybe because he is from the South, but I think that it happens here [in Turin] too. Even here in the North people take care of their parents, if they can. They take their parents home with them. . . . In other words, it's normal for him and for us.

Some families had sold both their previous home and the older person's home to buy a larger home that could accommodate them all. Most family members believe that keeping the older relative at home among their own things, among their memories, enabling them to maintain their habits and their routines, and above all to be surrounded by people who care for them is a sort of moral imperative that needs to be passed onto future generations. Benedetta, who cared for her 80-year-old mother together with her sister, explicitly reiterated these views:

> Every time I think that it is time to put her in a nursing home, I go to look at a few of them. Every time I've walked out crying, thinking "no, it's too

> early . . . we can still manage." Over these 10 years we've taken care of her with the help of at least 10 different home eldercare assistants. We did this because she's our mother and from a moral standpoint we believe that we should take care of her. Furthermore, my sister and I thought that it was important to set an example for our children, to show them that it is important to take care of your own elders, of your family.

Benedetta's words were echoed in most of the interviews, even if the reasons that drove the family members to keep their frail relatives either with them or in their own homes were diverse and in some cases conflicting. Among the reasons mentioned were affection, respect, gratitude, duty, guilt, and, last but not least, the fear of their own old age. Most families also believed that to place the older person in a residential facility would amount to consigning them to a depressing and lonesome environment that would hasten their mental decline. Arianna, who cared for her 89-year-old aunt, expressed such views cogently:

> When I first spoke with social services, they said that they could find me a place in a facility but my aunt was so used to being independent that I couldn't really agree to it. To dismantle her house, to put her in that facility that I have seen . . . and I'm not saying that they suffer there, no, but my aunt's mind is still fine, while some of the elders there are drooling or are grieving all the time. . . . I don't want my old age to be like that.

Other families instead were plainly concerned about the conditions experienced by the elders in some residential institutions. Piera, who with her sister Silvana cared for her frail mother, gave a particularly distressing account:

> We had a terrible experience with my mother-in-law. . . . She was in a facility where there were only two people to care for 15–20 elderly residents. . . . It looked pretty nice--they had their own cute, little room, but . . . . when the care-workers were busy and couldn't attend to them, or if an elder talked too much, they would tie them to their chairs, and we eventually figured out that my mother-in-law spent hours tied to her chair looking at a wall and she went crazy because of that . . . plus they kept men and women together and one of these men, he was sick I understand, but he gave her a beating and broke her nose, and nobody noticed for days. It was only when my mother-in-law was sent to the hospital that everything came out and we ended up filing a complaint with the police.

For others, the decision to keep a frail older parent at home and next to them was dictated not by a general fear of institutions but by the wish that they remain in their family's life, in other words to ensure that their relationship with their parents was a daily and close one, not one mediated by the schedule of an institution. Claudia candidly explained:

> I'm not necessarily against the institutions themselves. . . . Actually, I think that in recent years they have improved quite a bit . . . but I know that I would miss him, I would miss his presence. Being able to see him only during visiting hours, maybe only once a week or maybe even every day but amidst many people would not be enough, and I would miss him.

Moral, cultural, and traditional concerns, however, were not the only reasons that kept family members from placing their older relative in an institution; for some there was also the high cost. One son-in-law, Cosimo, explained the dilemma:

> I think that the current situation is a disaster, a disaster because there are not enough structures [residential facilities] for frail elders.[2] There aren't enough. For a residential home, a modest one, private for sure, one has to pay between 1,700 and 2,500 euros a month. My father-in-law's pension is 1,000 euros a month.[3] What can he do with 1,000 euros a month? Today to have a relatively self-sufficient elder in the family placed in an institution has become a luxury, something that most people cannot afford. I am not a privileged person but I'm not poor, I belong to the middle class, to the bourgeoisie. Well, I find myself in a situation in which both my wife and I work and we cannot afford to put my father-in-law in a residential facility.

The cost of residential facilities in Italy is indeed fairly high. The monthly fee at a *casa di riposo* [residential home care] for residents who are relatively self-sufficient or have low intensity care needs is on average €1,600, whereas the monthly fee at a nursing home may be as high as €2,000[4] (Altroconsumo, 2013; Lyon, 2006). According to a 2006 study conducted by the Osservatorio Terza Età/Aging Society only 5% of the elders who make use of residential services receive total coverage from the state. For 62% of those elders the costs of their stay fall upon themselves or their families, whereas in 33% of the cases the costs are partially covered by the national healthcare system (Osservatorio Terza Età/Aging Society, 2006; Polverini et al., 2004).[5]

Finally, admission to public residential institutions, which usually have lower costs, is not easy and in the Piedmont region an applicant is placed on a waiting list for at least 2 years (personal communication). The costs of hiring a home eldercare assistant are often no more than or lower than residential fees. Wages vary greatly, from €1,500 per month for a live-in worker with a residence permit to €450 per month for a live-in worker who has just entered the country without authorization (personal communication)—putting this kind of private arrangement in reach of even lower middle-class families (Glucksmann & Lyon, 2006).[6] Claudia told more of her personal accounting:

> To hire two full-time home eldercare assistants that rotate in order to provide 24-hour, seven days a week assistance while being able to take breaks and time off, I spend 1,700 euros a month plus room-and-board for both of them.[7] . . . We considered that from an economic standpoint the costs were more or less the same.

For all the reasons that have been mentioned, only four of the 28 interviewees expressed an active interest in pursuing the institutionalization of the elders in their care, and even in those cases it was a possibility for the future more than an active project.

FAMILY CAREGIVERS AND PUBLIC SERVICES: AN UNFRIENDLY RELATIONSHIP

Once the option of an institutional placement was discarded, the respondents believed that they had few choices apart from providing the care themselves or turning to the informal market of paid providers of care. This reflects the lack of information about public services. Most family members describe their contacts with social services as haphazard and not the outcome of a full and well-informed appraisal of their situation. Costanza, who with her sister cared for her mother, exemplified such experiences:

> We arrived at social services by chance, because we were looking for a residential facility for our mother and we were looking around. . . . Then one day we went to see a place in San Donato and the nuns there told us what to do, that we needed to have "a disability visit." From there on, various people told us other things and we kind of pieced it together.

Costanza's experience was similar to those of many of interviewed family caregivers. Many described their encounter with social services as a tortuous, difficult process frustrated by a lack of coordination among different institutions and a great deal of bureaucracy. Although public services and cash transfers for eldercare have slowly increased since the 1990s in Italy, the growth has been dispersed among different structures at different levels, from social services to the National Health Care System (NHCS), and among the states, regions, and municipalities. This lack of coordination has in turn created fragmented and dispersed knowledge about what is available, and a coherent picture rarely reaches the general public. For this reason, most families tend to rely on information that is disseminated through informal networks of friends, relatives, or work colleagues. Serafina, an octogenarian woman who cared for her 90-year-old sister, gave an account of the elusiveness of up-to-date information: "We heard of this possibility of assistance offered by the ASL (the local agency of the NHCS) through the son of a friend. . . . Well, his father who has now died got it and I think it would be really helpful for us, considering that I'm 82 and it's becoming harder and harder for me to take care of her." Furthermore, the lack of coordination among different institutions increased the time and energy that families had to spend before they could access a service, a cash transfer, or even just a wheelchair. Vilma eloquently complained:

> The most stressful aspect of dealing with the local agency of the National Health Care System and the social services is the bureaucracy; it kills everything. They presuppose that one has all the time in the world to spend running around from one office to another. It's a full-time job: how am I supposed to do it considering that I have my job to go to?

Additionally the long, extended waits caused by complex, multilevel application and assessment procedures were found to be inconsistent with the often urgent and serious conditions of the elders. Porzia, who cared for her 90-year-old mother, had been made distraught by the process:

> I say my mother is now 90 years old but if it was for the public services she would have been buried ten years ago. It is absolutely indecent. . . . They make you call a thousand times, and either the line is busy or they find a million excuses. They keep sending me from one place to the other while her health keeps deteriorating.

Things did not improve even after the family caregiver had overcome the initial difficulties and actually filed an official application. Many complained that the procedures for obtaining specific services were vague and intrusive, and that the final decision was based on the whim of the person in charge. Bettina, who cared for her mother suffering from Alzheimer's disease, described her experience:

> [Going through the social services] has been a strain; I took my mother to an appointment for claiming the *indennità di accompagnamento* [State Care Allowance][8] with all the required documents: cat scans, doctor's notes and so on and so forth, and they decided that she was only 70 percent disabled and therefore didn't deserve the allowance. I became really angry and said to the doctors, "What do you mean? What can she do with that 30%, how can she be alone?" And they said, "Sorry, Madam, this is the law." So, I waited some more time and presented the request again, more offices, more lines, and at the second visit they recognized

> her disability at a 100% and gave me the allowance and I asked, "What has changed from last time," but they didn't even bother answering me.

Finally, some family caregivers were upset by the discrepancy between the official discourse promoted by the NHCS and social services, which emphasizes the importance of keeping frail elders at home, and the actual support for families to make that possible, which they considered insufficient in terms of both services and cash transfers. Claudia dismissed the rhetoric with feeling:

> I don't know if you have seen in the newspapers, but everywhere they broadcast that it is better to keep the elders at home with their families. I say fine, I'll do it, even if I know that is a great saving for the community because the expenses for their care fall on us . . . but give us some help. A little something . . . they never gave me anything, either for my mother or my father. This famous *indennità di accompagnamento,* I have never seen it.

Social services, in fact, concentrate almost exclusively on extremely poor families, leaving others feeling helpless (Da Roit, 2007). Alberto related his experience:

> When we went to social services, they told us that they could have offered us some financial support if we had left my father in his own apartment, but now that we had taken him in, he is no longer eligible for that assistance. I don't know how this is possible, considering that in my family of four, I am the only one with an income and I'm a factory worker.

But even when the elders were living by themselves, the criteria for receiving public assistance were very strict. Costanza clarified this:

> When I went to social services to request some help to care for my mother, they asked me how much money my mother had in the bank, and because I don't know how to lie, I answered 15 million of old lire, her lifetime savings. The social worker said, "Well if she has that [amount] there is nothing we can do. We can provide something only when she has no more than €2,000 in her account." They will start to help her only when she has not even enough to pay for her own funeral.[9]

Lack of information, poor coordination among different public institutions, the extensive bureaucracy, the vagueness of procedures, and perhaps, most importantly, the fact that public services are directed only toward the most indigent families have generated a widespread sense of dissatisfaction and distrust toward the public care services and agencies. These sentiments tend to deter families, particularly the more affluent ones, from approaching social services at all. Maurizia, who supervised the care of her mother, declared: "No, [I never approached the] social services, because I knew that the help they could offer would have been less than what I needed." Not all families, however, could afford to forego financial assistance and 25 respondents interviewed for this project had applied for (but not necessarily obtained) one or more state benefits.[10] At the time of these interviews most families were still waiting to hear from social services, and had been waiting from 3 to 6 months, but most had already activated different channels to obtain help through the informal labor market. Most public provisions, with the exception of very limited homecare assistance directly provided by the social services, are cash transfers directly offered to the elders and their families that, while providing economic support, do not help them find home care workers. Many times during the participant observation, I observed family members who had taken their elderly relatives to the geriatric unit for a disability assessment ask social workers for a list of potential home eldercare assistants. The invariable answer was, "We are very sorry but we cannot provide this information here."[11] It is therefore understandable that families turn to the informal networks of friends, relatives, neighbors, and work colleagues for advice and information, and to the informal labor market to find home eldercare assistants.

HOW FAMILY CAREGIVERS BECOME EMPLOYERS

A much more immediate, effective, and flexible alternative to public services is offered by the informal labor market in which employers can purchase the help of im/migrant workers with little delay. Giulia, who cared for her husband with Alzheimer's disease, declares:

> I couldn't take it any longer. . . . I never asked anything of anybody, but at a certain point I understood that I couldn't do it any longer. I couldn't sleep more than three or four hours per night, so I thought, "I'll go to the office at the church" [to find help], and I did, I went there. . . . There were two elderly volunteers and I explained my problem to them. They looked at a list with the names of people who had recently come by asking for work.

Giulia's account illustrates the ways in which many of the interviewed family caregivers became employers. The decision to seek paid help, in fact, often emerged from an emergency, a breaking point that pushed family caregivers to find immediate help. The reasons behind this decision are many: for some, like Giulia, the main motives are fatigue and exasperation. For others it is the desire to delegate care, at least temporarily, to somebody else. Arianna explained:

> I can't wait to hear if the city is going to grant us some help with home eldercare assistance, I can't wait to delegate to somebody else, I don't care

> about the 400 euros,[12] as long as they will give me an amount that will allow me to go back to a normal life . . .

For some others the reason for turning to im/migrant women is the desire to find a full-time surrogate for themselves. Maurizia declared: "I didn't choose a person to care for my mother. I found one. . . . It was either she or I." Regardless of the reasons, most family members had reached a point of no return. For some, this decision came after years of extended care; for others, it was only after a few weeks; but when taken, it had an urgency that only the informal labor market seemed able to satisfy. This is why several families approached potential home eldercare assistants even before determining whether they would receive any economic support from the state,[13] choosing to use their own economic resources to cover the expenses. Cash transfers provided from the social services were, in fact, more often used to extend the hours of purchased care rather than trigger the initial arrangement.

The next obstacle described by the respondents was how to find the help they needed. As mentioned before, the state and public services did not provide any support in this sense, and therefore families relied mostly on word of mouth spread through informal networks. Quinto, a son caring for his father, explained:

> Well, I started by asking people I knew, word of mouth, because what can one do? First one goes to the church to see if there is a list, then one asks social services, then, what can one do? You can't find this kind of help in the yellow pages. Then a friend says: "Look I know a woman who. . ."

Quinto's experience was common among many family caregivers who become employers. They mentioned acquaintances, co-workers, and neighbors, and in some cases organizations such as the parish or Tierra, as their main source of information. Like the American employers of domestic workers described by Hondagneu-Sotelo (2001), most Italian family members are new to this experience; they never had to care for elderly parents in the past, let alone find somebody in the marketplace to care for their elders. Unlike child care or domestic jobs that have a history, eldercare is a new need, and often family members require the help of other people who went through similar experiences to navigate the situation.

The lack of formal recruiting, often the lack of a formal contract,[14] and the inexperience of both parties necessarily involve a great deal of trust. On the one hand, im/migrant workers need to trust employers for wages, for hours, for general living and working conditions, and sometimes, also for obtaining the necessary paperwork to gain legal status in the country. On the other hand, employers need to trust im/migrant workers to provide eldercare, but also to respect the privacy of their own home and their property. Honesty and reliability therefore are seen as the main requirements for this job, coming before any other ability or skill. To obtain these qualities, employers rely either on the experiences of other people in the same situation or on domestic and care workers who have already gained their trust. It is not uncommon for an employer to hire a person only because she is, supposedly, a friend or a relative of her current employee. Vanna stated:

> The woman who sleeps here at night to provide company to my mom is a relative of Giulia, the Romanian domestic worker I had for years. Her name is Danis. . . . I'm comfortable because I already know the family.

The same desire for reliability is what at times may provide migration opportunities to more than one woman in the same family. Arianna said:

> I met this Romanian lady in my building because she works for a company that cleans the stairs of my building and she offered to look after my aunt for a few hours a week, but she said that if we needed somebody for more hours she could call her daughter who is still back home.

The practice of hiring across national borders occurs primarily with Eastern European women, and is facilitated by geographic proximity,[15] but the practice is also seen with other ethnic groups who are considered *culturally* prone to care such as Filipinas and Latin American women (Andall, 2004; Zontini, 2002, personal conversations). This stress on the importance of reliability and dependability coupled with a growing number of im/migrant women available to perform these jobs is also generating a black market of eldercare services; im/migrant women who have greater access to jobs acquire these jobs with the sole purpose of selling them to other women who may be new to domestic work, may have just entered the country, or simply have more difficulties in finding a position (Mazzacurati, 2005, personal conversations).

Aside from trustworthiness and reliability, other qualities listed by the employers included patience, humanity, diplomacy, respectfulness, sensibility, attentiveness, kindness, and a loving attitude. The list shows that in these working relations there is always a blurring of the lines between the qualities strictly connected to the ability to perform the job and the personal qualities of the workers (Alemani, 2004; Anderson, 2001). Claudia explained:

> As an essential characteristic I would say that she would have to be available and profoundly human, because that is very important, I could not stand the idea of having a cold woman next to my father, somebody who does this job only to get the check at the end of the month, I could not stand it. These ladies who work for me, I must say, they really put all of themselves in this job and the elder perceives that, and I can see that my father is different now . . .

In some cases, the employers requested specific ethnicities, cultural backgrounds, and even levels of education. Orazio had a very particular profile of a desirable person to provide care:

> For me the person [who should care for my mother] should be sweet, sweet and obliging. . . . I don't know how to say it, maybe obliging is a bad term, but I think that she shouldn't be a Romanian, more like a Peruvian . . . . I say this because recently I have contacted a woman from Peru for my mother and she is a completely different person, maybe because they come from a different education, a less developed world and they are satisfied with less, they are more available, more kind. The Romanians instead feel more entitled, they don't think of themselves as domestic workers. . . .

Orazio's comments illustrate how racial, ethnic, national, educational, and class differences play a part in determining who is selected to provide care and how.

As pointed out by Parreñas (2001), choosing a worker who comes from a perceived poorer background and with lower education seems to guarantee a heightened predisposition for servitude and deference, characteristics that employers consider important not only for domestic workers but also for home eldercare assistants. In addition, choosing workers with such perceived characteristics helps to replicate the traditional relationship of domestic work in Italy, where caring and cleaning were historically the realm of women coming from rural areas (Sarti, 2004).

Not all employers, however, were as candid about race, ethnicity, class, and nationality. The majority of the interviewees did not mention them, hardly ever letting themselves utter more than a few confused sentences on the topic. This is not to say that these classifications are not a concern, because according to the informal mediators of the various nongovernmental organizations that I consulted, race, ethnicity, age, nationality, and familial status are very important to potential employers. Nevertheless, the employers I interviewed seemed uncomfortable about talking to me about the subject.

The potential homecare assistant's efficiency, experience, and training were not emphasized by the employers, who were more interested in the emotional component of the job than its practical aspects, even when the elders' ailments required specific skills. It is interesting to note that only the families employing Italian home eldercare assistants mentioned experience with complex ailments such as Alzheimer's disease as an important criterion. All the others focused more on the personal characteristics of the employee. As Maurizia, whose mother was in her mid-90s, explained:

> When I hired Irina, I wanted somebody who would care for my mother with affection, somebody that my mother would enjoy, who was intelligent enough to understand her needs and who had a glimpse of psychology . . .

> in other words my substitute. . . . The fact that she had been a nurse in the past was certainly a plus but not so much [important].

Although not all employers are as candid as Maurizia in explicitly stating that they are looking for a substitute for themselves in providing company and a presence for their parents and relatives, this idea is often implicit in their words and even in the characteristics they list. Most of these characteristics are usually connected to the notion of femininity: sweetness, loving attitude, humanity, and patience. For others, however, the cost of labor is what keeps them from hiring more qualified personnel. The socioeconomic background of the family and the amount of public aid the family receives deeply affect these choices (Bruno & Ugolini, 2013). Vanna clarifies:

> I can't afford it [to hire a nurse], I can't. . . . I tried to find a nurse to come in the morning to do what I do to my mother, clean her every morning. . . . I tried. I found this lady, a Romanian woman and she charged 8 euros[16] per hour and four more in the weekends. How can I afford that? I already have somebody to keep my mother company that costs me 650 euros[17] a month, then there is the other one who sleeps here with my mother, who I pay only a couple of hundred, plus room and board. I can't afford anything else.

The subcontracting of care duties to a substitute tended to create a great deal of anxiety and guilt among the family caregivers, to the point that even when the elders and the home eldercare assistants had established a harmonious relationship, most of the employers, specifically women, did not completely stop providing care. Even when they were affluent and were able to purchase all the hours of care that were needed, most family caregivers continued to supervise the care three or four times a week if not daily. Claudia gave a clear description of the complementary roles:

> Even now I go there first thing in the morning every day, to check how he [her father] passed the night. . . . After that, I make sure that he still has all the medicines he needs, because I'm the one still in charge of this aspect. I go to the doctor, I go to the pharmacy, I take care of all the requests that need to go through the health care system or the social services, like a visit to a specialist or getting a special pillow, a special mattress. I ask the women what they need and I procure it for them. The assistants take care of the daily needs like groceries, newspapers and so on.

Such "management of care" was, however, almost exclusive to the upper-class families in which hiring a home eldercare assistant not only provided a hands-on care provider but was also an active substitution for some aspects of psychosocial care. In these cases, as Romero (1992, p. 131) pointed out, the employers want help with more than the manual tasks; they expect psychological needs to be met and their own self-esteem and well-being to be enhanced (cf. Ayalon, 2009). Employers achieve these goals by supervising and monitoring the employee's work, which elevates their feelings of power and authority. The change from a caregiver to a care-manager also allows the employer to maintain moral and spiritual control over the health and the well-being of the elders, which enables the traditional family role to persist and the relative's reputation as a responsible, filial caring person to be largely sustained.

CONCLUSIONS

The in-depth interviews analyzed in this chapter provide important insight into the current eldercare regime operating in Italy and supply a snapshot of the complex interplay among families, the state, and the market. In addition, the words of the family caregivers provide a deeper understanding of the meanings that family caregivers attribute to their own and paid carers' roles and on the reasons that bring them to become employers of immigrant workers. Although not generalizable to the rest of the population, the small sample confirms the result of other studies (among others Bettio & Verashchagina, 2010) indicating that the majority of long-term care continues to be provided by women and that even when men are present, there continues to be a gendered division of labor, according to which women provide and manage the actual care while men provide support by bringing the elders to doctors' visits or dealing with the bureaucracy of public aid. In addition, it contributes a deeper understanding of the needs that long-term care generates. The interviews indicate that the reasons why Italian women, and to a lesser extent Italian men, hire home eldercare assistants are complex and are not simply influenced by economic reasoning but also by cultural and ethical considerations. First, the presence of immigrant women in Italy allows Italian families to provide personalized and individualized care for their elders—at a cost lower than the cost of most residential facilities, which places home eldercare in reach of even lower middle-class families. Second, it provides families with the ability to uphold a model of care that is rooted in cultural, social, and moral traditions. The model that has become established considers families, and particularly women, as the key providers of family care, discourages institutionalization, and favors keeping frail older people in their own homes and among their possessions, memories, and families.

Third, the presence of immigrant women allows family caregivers of all social classes to shift their position from "care providers" to "care managers." The change in role allows Italian caregivers to delegate the most demeaning aspects of long-term care while retaining moral and spiritual control over the health and the well-being of their relative, thus allowing them to fulfill the traditional filial role. In other words, the work of im/migrant women allows Italian families and the Italian welfare state to maintain the status quo and to continue to function without having to conceptualize new or alternative models of care. Immigrant women workers provide not only flexible and often poorly paid labor, but also, to a degree, perpetuate a normative model of the caring family both at a private and at an institutional level. Fourth, the support that immigrant women provide to Italian family caregivers allows the Italian welfare state not only to save money by delegating more and more of the care into the hands of families as mentioned in Chapter 3 (shorter hospital stays, encouraging people to keep elders at home), but, perhaps most importantly, also to avoid a rediscussion and radical restructuring of the obsolete and inflexible *familialistic* model. The interviews, in fact, provide meaningful insight into Italian attitudes toward the welfare state and the private-care market. Although the wealthiest respondents had a clear preference for the free market and wished to bypass the state, the majority wanted the welfare state to play a stronger role in and to provide more help in navigating the increased burden of long-term eldercare. In most cases, the decision to turn to the market came only after all other options had been exhausted. The respondents provided a clear message indicating that Italian families long for a restructured welfare state that offers them not only financial assistance, but perhaps, most importantly, much better information, services, and support.

ACKNOWLEDGMENTS

Material in Chapter 4 is adapted from Francesca Degiuli, "The Burden of Long-Term Care: How Italian Family Care-Givers Become Employers." *In Ageing and Society*, 30(5), July 2010, 755–777, Cambridge Journals.

NOTES

1 Approximately US $608.
2 Public residential facilities in the Turin area have a waiting list of a minimum of 2 years, while financial support to access the private sector homes is offered only to people who declare very low income (Polverini et al., 2004, p. 59).
3 The equivalent in US dollars are, respectively, $1,915–2,815 and $1,126.
4 €1,100–1,200 is approximately US $1,228–$1,340.
5 According to the website of the Region Piemonte, expenses concerning the residential structures are distributed as follows: the room and board expenses are paid by the elders or their families, whereas the medical expenses are paid by the National Health Care System. If the income of the

elders and their families is below a certain amount (including not only yearly income but also all personal property) the municipality will provide some financial support. http://www.provincia.torino.it/sportellosociale/anziani/sa11

6 Approximate equivalent are US $1,690 and $507.

7 Approximate equivalent is US $1,916.

8 The *indennità di accompagnamento* [State Care Allowance] is described in detail in Chapter 3.

9 15 million old lire is approximately US $10,000 and €2,000 is approximately US $2,706.

10 The most frequently applied for benefits were *assistenza domiciliare* [Homecare Assistance], the *assegno di cura* [Care Allowance], *affidamento famigliare* [Family Reimbursement Cheque], and the *indennità di accompagnamento* [State Care Allowance]. All of these cash allowances are described in detail in Chapter 3.

11 This has changed in recent years particularly in larger cities as will be discussed in Chapter 8, but not everywhere in the country.

12 Approximately US $450.

13 Cash transfers provided from the social services are often more of a means to extend the hours of care that families can purchase than the main reasons why families buy care services.

14 Ironically, Italy is one of the few countries that has a national contract that regulates care and domestic work, a contract that was renewed in March 2007. The new contract implies eight different levels of qualification and wages. It regulates the maximum number of hours that both live-in and live-out workers can work a week, establishes the amount of paid leave, vacation, and sick days that the workers can receive, and establishes the rest that they need to receive daily, particularly in the case of live-in workers. Unfortunately, however, only documented im/migrant workers with formal arrangements can benefit from this contract. All irregular workers and those hired under informal arrangements do not.

15 As a matter of fact, not so much in Torino, but particularly in the Northeast of Italy it is common to hear about Eastern European women who practice *pendulum migration* meaning that they enter the country either through a tourist visa or their EU status, work in Italy for 4 or 6 months as live-in eldercare assistants, and then go back home while being replaced by a close relative for the other 6 months (Bettio et al., 2006).

16 Approximately US $9 dollars.

17 The equivalent of US $732 dollars.

5
THE SHAPING OF NEW SUBJECTS

> "Cerco seconda badante fissa per anziana non autosufficiente, lavoro con altra badante italiana già presente, necessarie pazienza, adattabilità, esperienza, meglio se con referenze, gentilezza di carattere, capacità di gestire la casa, cucinare, ecc." (07/22/2014 www.kijiji.it n.68247714)

> "Seeking second badante (home eldercare assistant) to care for a non self-sufficient elder, the person will have to share the work with another Italian badante already present, characteristics needed: patience, adaptability, experience, possibly with previous references. Also required: kindness, ability to manage the house, cook, etc." (ad number 68247714v placed on 07/22/2014 on www.kijiji.it)

As the ad above and the words of the Italian employers in the previous chapter show, perspective employers have very specific ideas of who they would like to hire to provide care for their elders. The question that follows then is do im/migrant women actually embody the ideal employee that Italian employers seek? Or, rather, are they transformed to fit this mold? In this chapter I argue that im/migrant women do not necessarily fit the mold of the "ideal home eldercare assistant"; rather they are *transformed into it* through a number of different processes that go from global to local and from public to private. In the previous chapter I argued that the lack of public services coupled with an increase in cash for care allowances and public pensions have encouraged Italian families to seek help for their long-term needs in the market. This market, however, is not a fully developed institution and very few private enterprises[1] have started to develop in this area. The result is that the market available to Italian families remains for the most part an informal market made up of individuals who sell their services directly to families. In the previous chapter I explored how Italian families turn into employers and the ways in which these new employers approach and select *home eldercare assistants.* In this chapter, instead, I will investigate how im/migrant women are transformed into the workers needed by Italian families and, by extension, by the Italian state. Im/migrant women do not always magically appear in the countries of the Global North to fulfill a specific labor market niche, rather they are channeled into it through a variety of practices and discourses. The majority of the immigrant women I interviewed for this project declared that they had no experience in taking care of elders and some of them had no previous experience in domestic work. Some knew that they were coming to engage in this specific occupation, but many others had very different expectations at the inception of their migratory journey. Nevertheless, in a matter of days or months, these women, independent of their countries of origin, or their backgrounds in terms of race, ethnicity, class, education, and nationality, were transformed into home eldercare assistants. In this chapter I explore the different stages of this transformation both at the global and at the local level and, because every niche of the economy is culturally shaped (Tsing, 2005), I explore how Italian employers construct and adhere to hierarchies of race, ethnicity, nationality, family status, and age to create the ideal home eldercare assistant.

THE CREATION OF NEW SUBJECTS

Im/migrant women coming to Italy from countries as diverse as Romania, Peru, Nigeria, and the Philippines have very different class, educational, and professional backgrounds. Some of these women grew up poor whereas others found themselves in economic difficulties only after political and socioeconomic developments such as the collapse of the Soviet Union or the expansion of neoliberal ideologies in developing countries. Some came from rural families of very modest means, whereas others came from professional families employing domestic workers. Some are highly educated with Ph.D.s in engineering, architecture, and medicine, whereas others only finished grade school. Yet independently from their class and their educational and professional backgrounds, once they enter Italy im/migrant women are stripped of their knowledge, their education, their skills, and their histories. Madeline, a Congolese worker, explains:

> When a person enters Italy as a migrant worker she loses everything. They tell you that you are nothing... they even take away your knowledge, your education, your professional experience.

In the migration process women from the Global South and from post communist countries are deprived of their former identities and become part of a single group: im/migrant women. This status often overshadows the significance of other identities (Pojmann, 2006, p. 38) and allows for the creation of new subjects. Subjects are then redesigned according to the needs of the state, the families, and Italian society at large—an effect that in recent years has evolved into the designing of home eldercare assistants. To understand how this process came into place, it is crucial to try to understand who the home eldercare assistants desired by Italian families, and by extension by the Italian welfare state, are. A possible definition, according to my understanding of it, would read as follows:

> Home eldercare assistants are, for the most part, women who, in exchange for wages, provide the equivalent of a paid *traditional woman*,[2] whose life is dedicated, without either reservations or time limitations, to the house and the well-being of the elders.

According to the majority of the people interviewed for this project, eldercare work is made up of two inextricably related functions. On the one hand, it provides productive work geared to satisfying the basic needs involved in reproduction. It supplies food and its preparation, cleanliness of the house, hygiene of the elder, emotional and psychological support, and, in many cases, also some basic nursing skills. On the other hand, it allows for the reproduction of an ideal familial arrangement, that of the extended family, which no longer exists in contemporary post industrial societies. The presence of im/migrant women working as home eldercare assistants does not provide employers necessarily with a better lifestyle, with higher status, or with the possibility of better and/or higher paid careers as is the case with domestic workers and nannies (Anderson, 2001; Näre, 2012; Yeates, 2009). Rather it provides them with a chance to create a *fictional extended family*, one in which women perceived as less fortunate and from, supposedly, less developed countries are given the task to keep alive ideal notions of gender roles and family that, due to demographic, economic, social, and cultural changes, no longer exist (McDonald, 2011; Parreñas, 2014). As Vaifre Palanca, a im/migrant woman who worked for the Italian Commission of Political Integration of Immigrants, pointedly stated:

> Immigrant women [in Italy] are reconfirmed in their traditional role as custodians of family values and as links to home culture. This is a role that is carried on in a domestic intimacy and is reinforced thorough contact with other women (1999, p. 109).[3]

In the Italian case the practice of treating care workers as "one of the family," a practice extensively described in the literature on domestic work (among others Bettio, Simonazzi, & Villa, 2006; McDonald, 2011; Parreñas, 2014), reflects not just a way to incorporate the immigrant worker into the structure of the family in order to extract more labor, justify lower wages (Romero, 2002), or create a stronger attachment to the elders, rather, it reflects the need to recreate an organizational structure essential to the functioning of Italian society. The re-creation of this structure is functional not only to Italian families that do not have to envision new social arrangements or challenge the traditional gendered division of labor (Andall, 2000; Lyon, 2006), but also to the Italian welfare state that due to this internal reorganization of the family does not have to restructure itself. The familialist regime that characterizes the Italian welfare state can continue to function as long as the majority of care continues to be provided by families or their proxy (Bettio et al., 2006). The presence of im/migrant women workers therefore allows the perpetuation of a fictional reality both at the private and the institutional level. In addition, this perpetuation is achieved at low cost, because, as seen in Chapter 3, taking care of the elders at home with the help of home eldercare assistants is often cheaper than placing them in residential facilities. These low costs can be further reduced by hiring irregular workers or workers who engage in circular migration and who are not interested in being hired formally. According to sociologist Costanzo Ranci (2002), hiring an irregular worker or a regular migrant in an informal arrangement allows families to save between 30% and 50% of the costs of a native or regular immigrant. Employers save on social security contributions, holiday/vacation pay, overtime, and the end of contract settlement,[4] while the welfare state saves on health-related costs, nursing facilities, and targeted services.

THE IDEAL HOME ELDERCARE ASSISTANT

As mentioned in the introduction, although a few im/migrant women enter the country already knowing that they will work as home eldercare assistants, the majority of them enter this occupation only because of a lack of better opportunities (Bettio et al., 2006; Da Roit & Facchini; 2010; Fullin & Vercelloni, 2009). Beatriz, a Peruvian worker, points out:

> In Peru I used to work for a consulting firm; a company would give us a building project and we would help them to make it happen. When I came to Italy I certainly didn't expect to find the same job, but at the same time I had no idea that I would end up working as a home eldercare assistant. When Pilar [the TierraMadre cultural mediator] offered me the job I was utterly terrified, particularly of the domestic aspect of it. I never had to clean or to cook before, I don't know how to do it and, in truth, I never liked it. Nevertheless now I can manage.

As Beatriz's words emphasize, the women and men who would neatly fit the definition of home eldercare assistants do not really exist. Like the Los Angeles-based care and domestic workers described by Hondagneu-Sotelo (2001) and the British domestic workers examined by Anderson (2000), home eldercare assistants in Italy are *made* both at the state level through migration laws but also through preconceived notions, stereotypes, and daily practices enforced from different social actors. Drawing on the work of both Hondagneu-Sotelo (2001) and Anderson (2000), in this chapter I explore how employers and the informal mediators of Benevolentia, Tierra, and Apidad help to create the *ideal* home eldercare assistant through discourses and the construction of different hierarchies of race, ethnicity, nationality, age, and familial status. The creation of these temporary family members to support or substitute for Italian women in the provision of care happens at different levels: global and local and private and public, in a convergence of historical and new elements that only in its last stage directly implicates the families and the workers themselves.

The creation of ideal workers starts with the social representation of immigrants by the mass media, the government, and society at large. In Italy, as in most other postindustrial countries including the United States, im/migrant workers are either presented negatively as usurpers, as potential competitors for jobs and public services, as criminals, or, and this is the position usually adopted by the Catholic Church and some sectors of the left, as "people in need who come here to do the jobs that Italians no longer want." Although these two positions are a generalization of the more complex attitudes that Italians have toward im/migrant women and men, they tend to capture two main discourses used to define *foreigners* in Italy. In a way, these positions repeat the scheme illustrated by Simmel (1908/1971) according to which the foreigner can be perceived either as a *barbarian* or something *other*—potentially dangerous—and at the same time *one of us*, not exactly like us but part of a general community, of humanity at large.

Mass media, in particular, are responsible for amplifying this dichotomy (Cotesta, 2002). First, they produce extensive daily reports on crimes committed by different ethnic groups, or alternatively, but certainly less often, they focus on how important im/migrant work is for the functioning of the Italian economy. These depictions of im/migrant workers and of their presence in Italy are coupled with a persistent portrayal of most of the developing world and post communist countries as *other*: as poor, underdeveloped, and backward. Pilar, a Peruvian cultural mediator, says:

> When they show our countries on TV, the Third World in general, they always show poverty; that's the only thing they show.... For this reason most people in Italy think that we are savages.... When they give us a job they control our food, they treat us as slaves, they do not think of us as people like them.

Such portrayals result in the creation of distance between Italian citizens and im/migrant workers—a distance created not only by visible differences, as in the case of race and ethnicity, but also by marked cultural differences (Balibar, 1988, 1991; Taguieff, 1987, 2001) that work as proxies for biologically grounded racial categories. As Paul Gilroy (2004, p. xv) points out, *cultural racism* has substituted the previously biologically based racism. Racist claims in contemporary societies are hidden under assertions of "civilizational differences" so that "the convenient argument that some cultural differences are so profound that they cannot be bridged has become commonplace." These cultural boundaries become then reified and naturalized in daily discourses (Pagliai, 2013, p. 49).

Im/migrant women in Italy, with the exception of sex workers who are criminalized (Pojmann, 2006), tend to fall in the second category—less fortunate people in need. Employers in some cases even tend to decouple them from the rest of the im/migrant population. Madeline recounts:

> One day my employer was reading the newspaper regarding an article on micro-criminality in the city and said loudly while I was in the other room tending to her mother, "These Moroccans and these Blacks. . .What are they doing here? What do they want from us?" I was shocked. . . . I looked at him and said, "Tomorrow I'm not coming to work because you insulted me and my identity both as an immigrant and as a Black." He looked at me as if he saw me in that light for the first time and said, "No, no . . . I wasn't talking about you; you are different."

In addition, im/migrant women in Italy do not often appear in sensationalist newspaper articles, and even less do they compete for jobs in traditional workplaces (Ambrosini, 2013; Giorgi, 2012). For the most part, instead, they tend to disappear behind the walls of private homes away from the public gaze. Their presence in the innermost private fabric of Italian families is not seen as an "invasion," a term often used to describe immigrant presence in the country, but rather as a continuation of the traditional structure of domestic work, historically fulfilled by poorer and lesser educated women coming first from rural areas of Italy and later from countries such as Eritrea, the Philippines, the Cape Verde Islands, Salvador, Somalia, and Sri Lanka, often thanks to the intermediation of the Church. This is also due to the fact that im/migrant women, even when educated, are not always able to have their diplomas or certifications recognized in the country in which they find work. In fact, even when legally possible, the amount of paperwork and bureaucracy involved in the process often discourages workers who are already struggling to learn a new language and negotiate a new country (personal conversations).

Being described as good people in need, however, is apparently only slightly less damaging than being criminalized. The notion of need acts as a powerful tool in creating a stigmatized and devalued workforce. Workers who are in need do not have the same rights as regular workers since jobs offered to people in need do not have the same qualities as regular jobs. Often employers think that merely by providing a job they are doing the prospective employee a favor, and because of that employers feel that they are exonerated from paying those employees livable wages, offering them decent working conditions, and respecting their basic rights, including holidays, sick days, maternity leave, and so on (Scrinzi, 2004). Vanna, for example, explains:

> I have two Romanian women who work for me. The first one I have hired, she has a contract, I pay taxes and everything, the second one, however, I do not pay. She comes only at night. She sleeps here and she works as a domestic during the day... I am giving her a place where to sleep every night. Yes, my mother keeps her awake sometimes... but when she bothers her too much she comes and get me... it's not as if she is really working.

THE BURDEN OF NEED

Im/migrant women in Italy are burdened by different layers of needs—the first of these due to their position in a global system of racial, class, and gender inequalities. Im/migrant workers *need* a job to live, to send remittances home, to have a place to stay, to make sense of their being migrants who have left their families and community of origin. This need is created at a macrolevel by global political economic and cultural processes that make women move away from their countries of origins. Esther, a Nigerian woman in her late 20s that came to Tierra to find a job, vents: "I feel like I have a fire burning inside me because for two months I haven't been able to send money to my son. What am I doing here if I'm not making money?... I have no reasons at all." Im/migrant women, particularly those who had to leave their families behind to migrate, need a job not only to earn wages but to make sense of their decision to leave. As Esther's words emphasize, obtaining a job and consequently being able to send remittances home helps to justify to their children, families, and communities their decision to challenge gender roles, become the breadwinner of the family, and forego their duties as mothers, daughters, and wives. Therefore, for im/migrant women the need to find a job has an urgency unparalleled among other groups of workers.

The need for work inherent to the migration project is often compounded by the debt accumulated in order to be able to migrate. Most women already arrive in the country with debts usually ranging from $1,500 to $2000 for women who live in Eastern Europe to $5,000 to $7,000 for women who have to travel overseas (personal communication). Very often in order to be able to start sending money home they have to repay the debt, and they have to do it quickly because the interest on the debt acquired tends to grow fast. Almira, a home eldercare assistant from Romania, explains:

> When we left we thought that we would come here to improve our lives, because we needed money to care for our children. . . but once we got here we saw what was available [job wise]. . . but it did not matter because to come we had to borrow money and therefore we had to work.

The need generated through the migration process is then further intensified by the need generated at the local level through immigration and citizenship laws. The current legislation, the Bossi-Fini law, more than previous legislations, ties im/migrant women and men exclusively to their function as workers. As shown in Chapter 3 (Table 3.3), migrants are allowed to stay in the country only as workers. Residency permits are granted only for a maximum of 2 years and renewals must be requested 3 months before expiration even if the worker has an open-ended contract. If, at the time of renewal, the worker does not have a job, she or he will be offered a 6-month grace period to find another job, but after that no further renewal will be granted and the im/migrant will have to leave the country.

The association established by the immigration law between work and im/migrant status keeps workers under the constant threat of losing their job or of having to find a new one. This fear was repeated constantly in the interviews. The need created by the state consequently forces im/migrant workers to take whatever job is available independent of the elders' physical and mental conditions, the hours, the working conditions, or the wages. Caterina Zamboni of Apidad, reports:

> Workers hoping to obtain the residency permit take everything; they suffer all sorts of abuse. Then when they obtain it, they want revenge. They come to the association with notes and notes on how much overtime they did, the holidays they worked and that were never paid double, but then it's too late and there is nothing we can do.

Finally, the constant need for work is exacerbated by the constant competition among new waves of im/migrant workers coming from different countries. As mentioned in Chapter 3, overtime changes in the structure of the European Union have simplified access for many migrants from Eastern Europe who are now able to come and go as they please, creating, at times, waves that overwhelm the market. All the mediators at the different organizations commented on how, at times, it could be difficult to find new jobs and how, at times, the supply by far surpassed the demand. Often, while observing Pilar at Tierra during the weekly meeting dedicated to women looking for care jobs, I noticed that she did not have jobs to offer, and when she did they were very demanding jobs requiring full time, live-in assistance to extremely disabled elders. The demand for employees was so low that for each job Pilar would introduce to prospective families and their elders three different women, different in terms of age, race/ethnicity, and personality, in order to provide them with the best match. Sister Ortensia speaks of similar difficulties at Benevolentia:

> The new amnesty (2003) and family reunification have allowed for the entrance of many new migrants and this has changed the work situation. There aren't that many jobs available anymore. The only requests we had for the past few weeks were for full-time live-in positions and not many people can take those. They need to be really desperate.

The large number of women available for these jobs in turn allows employers and mediators to enforce hierarchies of race/ethnicity, nationality, age, and familial status. Giulia's recollection of the selecting process is a good example of employers' power in designing the *ideal* employee:

> One day, when I couldn't take it any longer. I went to my church and in the office there were two elderly volunteers and I explained to them my situation. They looked at their list of recent arrivals and said "Here we have three women who really need work" and I said "Fine, but tell me their situation, are they married? Do they have kids?" And the lady answered, "Yes, this one has a toddler," and I said, "Then, no, it wouldn't work, because with a toddler we would always have trouble, I need a certain schedule and with a kid, it can't happen. What if he catches the flu? No. no." The lady then looked again and said, "We also have a woman of color here who would be available. She works in the office next door," and I said, "Sure if she speaks Italian well enough," but then something wasn't clear, like she already had half a job so I said, "Do you have anybody else?" And the lady said, "Well, there is this lady. She came today, she is married, she lives nearby." And I said, "Oh she lives close by, does she have kids? How old is she?" and the lady said "No, no kids, she is 34 years old," and at that moment I knew she was the one, I asked for her number and once home I called her and set up an appointment. She came after half an hour and I liked her a lot because she had a beautiful smile and she looked very sweet.

The above quote provides a snapshot of how selective employers of home elder-care assistants can afford to be, and how they often privilege immigrant workers personal qualities over their actual skills.

THE ENCOUNTER WITH THE EMPLOYERS

Once im/migrant women reach the doors of prospective employers they are no longer their former selves. Stripped of their education and knowledge, and burdened with multiple layers of need, im/migrant women can no longer present themselves as competent and professional workers but often simply as women "with a beautiful smile, looking sweet" joining the ranks of what MacDonald and Sirianni (1996) have defined as "emotional proletariat"—workers for whom self-presentation and other personal characteristics are seen as core job requirements (Stacey, 2011, p. 9). As seen in Chapter 4, in only a very few cases do Italian family caregivers look for professional eldercare workers to provide care for their elders and when they do they hire Italian workers for these positions. In the majority of cases, instead, employers seek the equivalent of what they think *a traditional woman* should be: a woman whose skills are *natural* ones, bestowed upon her by her gender, culture, nationality, and age. The most common requirements expressed by employers, in fact, do not reflect skills or abilities but simply personal qualities. Home eldercare assistance, in fact, is considered by most employers a *low-quality* (Wrigley, 1995) job because it is a *natural* job, one that all women know how to do on the basis of their gender and essentialized notions of what being a women means in other cultures (Parreñas, 2014). Employers often draw on stereotypical notions of femininity that portray women coming from other countries as "dutiful daughter, mother, wives raised in cultures emphasizing respect for the elders" (Chang, 2000, p. 113). According to the Italian caregivers I have interviewed, prospective employees have to be patient, good-natured, "have a nice smile," be respectful, and, perhaps most importantly, be available at all times for reasonable wages. In home eldercare assistance, and often in domestic work, employers buy more than a worker, they buy the whole personhood (Anderson, 2001), because what they are looking for is not really a worker but somebody who can potentially act as a less fortunate member of the family, albeit for a limited amount of time. The encounter with the employers, in other words, becomes the last stage in the process of subordination and devaluation of im/migrant workers.

In addition, it is in the encounter with employers and with cultural mediators, who enforce the requests of employers, that im/migrant women from the Global South and post communist countries lose their blanket status of *im/migrant woman* to be differentiated according to hierarchies of race and ethnicity, age, familial status, and more. Employers use stereotypes, preconceived notions about race and ethnicity, anecdotal experiences, and hearsay to find the help needed in the shortest amount of time, creating and reproducing stigmatizations and hierarchies very difficult for immigrant workers to escape (Cominelli, 2003).

As mentioned in the previous chapter, although the employers I interviewed very rarely expressed notions related to race and ethnicity, my participant observation at Tierra and the conversations with the operators and cultural mediators at Apidad, Benevolentia, and Tierra revealed that employers do construct and adhere to hierarchies of race/ethnicity, nationality, age, and familial status. These hierarchies in turn affect which women will get the best jobs and which women will get the most demanding and less remunerative ones (see among others Andall, 2000; Hondagneu-Sotelo, 2001; Scrinzi, 2004; Wrigley, 1995).

Italian employers tend to use nationality and the *type* of personality they ascribe to it to choose the employee that will best provide the service they need. When talking about their employees they often say, "I have a Peruvian who comes in the morning," or "I have a Romanian who provides care for my aunt," referring to their employees exclusively in terms of their nationality. This language shows how in Italy, as in the rest of Europe, employers of domestic and care workers tend to utilize what Anderson (1997, p. 46) calls a *pick and mix* racism to choose prospective employees, which results in the creation of hierarchies in the eldercare labor market. Furthermore, when asked why they employed a specific im/migrant worker instead of another, most of the employers provided answers such as "Peruvians have a culture of care," or "Filipinos are very respectful of the elders," indicating, as Gerd Baumann pointed out, that cultural differences have been naturalized in the dominant discourse and that attributed cultural characteristics have been reified into something that people *have* (Baumann, 1996; Pagliai, 2013). This practice is so common and widespread that im/migrant women themselves have learned how to use the notion of *culture* to gain the favor of employers over other workers. When asked what makes her good at her job, Hilda, a Filipino woman who has worked as a home eldercare assistant for more than 7 years, explains:

> Our (Filipino) culture teaches us to work with the heart, I think that this is key. We respect the elders and we love them. I behave with the elders here as I would behave at home. We kiss them, we cuddle them as we would do with our own elders at home, we give them love because this is what they need.

In some cases they even present themselves as "women who still know how to care" in contraposition to Italian families. Hilda continues:

> I understand that the sons and daughters now they have their lives... but my lady needs them... when I started working for her, I told her children "during the weekend you have to watch your mom. She is your mom, you have to take care of her... don't just give the job to me because I am a foreigner."

HIERARCHIES OF LABOR

According to my year-long participant observation at Tierra and what emerged from the interviews with both the employers and the employees, hierarchies of labor change depending on the availability of workers and the desires and need of the employers. During the late 1990s and early 2000s, women from Peru and the Philippines were among the most sought after workers both in terms of domestic and care work (Bettio et al., 2006). Among the many reasons that were cited, two were the most common: first their religious allegiance (both migrant groups are mostly Catholic), and second, most of the employers considered Peruvian and Filipino women better predisposed for care, because as Belinda, one of the employers, says, "People coming from these countries respect their elders more." Ligaya, a Filipino worker, explains:

> Italians, for some reason, really like us, the Filipinos, especially the elders do. They always say that we are good, honest, and that we smile all the time. They always get very emotionally attached to us.

Ligaya's words are confirmed by studies such as the ones by Chell-Robinson (2000) and Parreñas (2001). Chell-Robinson (2000, p. 109) states that in Italy, *Filipina* and *domestic worker* are synonyms in the Italian spoken language and that employers considered Filipina women the "domestic of preference," while Parreñas (2001, p. 178) indicates that Filipino workers in Italy claim to be the Mercedes Benz of domestic work. Filipino workers, however, are not interested in home eldercare positions because as Luzvminda, a home eldercare assistant and the president of the Filipino Catholic Association in Turin, clarifies: "People of my ethnic group work as home eldercare assistants only to get a foothold in this country because this job has no future."

This same notion is confirmed by the report compiled by the trade unionist, Carolina Cardenas (1998, p. 5): "Filipino workers are very professional and they aim at the higher positions of domestic work. Peruvian workers, instead, specialize in care jobs. This is why, at least in Turin, Peruvian women, and in some cases, Peruvian men, occupy the higher levels of the home eldercare labor market, often obtaining the best and better paid jobs."

The same level of appreciation is often shared by women of Central and South America, who, like Filipino and Peruvian women, are considered good nurturers and therefore apt to care for the elders. Italian employers seem to agree that women coming from this geographic area share a value system closer to the Mediterranean one, and therefore will not challenge the values, traditions, and habits of the elders. Additionally, as already pointed out in Chapter 4, workers coming from this geographic area are considered more deferential, more respectful, and more willing to accept difficult working conditions for lower wages than women from other geographic areas.

Eastern European women are another group that has a sizable presence in home eldercare assistance. Their participation in this occupation has been growing in recent years because as the last group to enter the country, they are often willing to accept, at least in the beginning, lower wages and the most demanding live-in positions. Nevertheless, Eastern European women, while potentially being advantaged by the color of their skin and by their cultural background as Europeans, did not necessarily represent the ideal employee, particularly in the early phase of this phenomenon. Employers described them as too bossy, too demanding, or too knowledgeable of their rights. Caterina Zamboni explains:

> The new immigration [the one from Eastern Europe] is a very aggressive migration; they know their rights very well but not their duties. Eastern Europeans have a better sense of what they can obtain as workers and they demand it. . . . They are aware of class disparities, and because of their history, less willing than others to accept them.

According to the words of the employers and the mediators, Eastern European women, because of their socialist background and therefore their longer experience in the labor market and their higher awareness of workers' rights, tend to scare employers looking for labor that is not only cheap, but also deferential and pliable to their needs.[5] When describing the ideal employee, in fact, employers concur in describing somebody who is able to perform only what they perceive as the basic elements of care: cleaning, feeding, medicating, and keeping company. Benedetta elucidates:

> For the time being, I don't need somebody with specific skills; what I need is somebody who will keep my mom clean, cared for, in a clean house. My sister and I are there for more complex things.

From the quote it is clear that although employers are willing to defer the most menial tasks of care, they are not willing to relinquish their role as supervisors of care and for these reasons they feel threatened by Eastern European workers who tend to take a more independent role in their approach to home eldercare work.

Furthermore, it is important to keep in mind that the tight bonds that the close quarters of home eldercare assistance generate between the elders and the im/migrant women who care for them constantly endanger Italian women's position as the *woman of the house* (padrona di casa).[6] Maurizia explains:

> The woman who works for me, she is good, she loves my mother, but like all the others . . . uhm . . . she loves her but she has become the one

> who rules here, like when she goes out ... my mother has a perfume that is no longer sold in stores and that can be found only in Paris, so my ex-husband who lives there buys it for her.... Well, today when I came in Irina had it on ... and I thought this is not good.... I had to tell her and then you know she lives here with her daughters... I mean I allowed her to do it but I need to come once in a while to make sure that my mother doesn't feel like she is no longer the person in charge here ... you know ... I don't want my mother to feel that she has lost her role as the woman of the house.

The struggle for power mentioned by Maurizia becomes even harder when the elders and the employers face workers more similar to them in terms of physical appearances, class background, and level of education, as in the case of Eastern European women.[7] Racialized difference, in fact, ensures a *safe* distance between employer and employee, or the elders and the employee (Bott, 2005), which in the case of Eastern European women is violated. This is why, notwithstanding their willingness to accept lower wages and live-in positions, Eastern European women are not necessarily at the top of the eldercare labor hierarchy, showing that cheap wages and compliance in accepting difficult working conditions are not the only elements that cause Italian employers to hire im/migrant workers.

Certainly there are exceptions to these rules and it is important to keep in mind that the immigrant experience of Eastern European women in Italy is not uniform. Whereas Romanian women are highly valued because of their ability to learn the language due to similarities between Italian and Romanian and because they can legally work in the country, Albanian women are highly discriminated against. Albanians, in fact, are one of the most feared groups in terms of criminality, and, therefore, the women of this ethnic group are generally at the bottom of the occupational hierarchy together with African women. Afrodita recounts:

> At the beginning I couldn't find any job, because as soon as they heard that I was from Albania, they would freeze. Inevitably the day after they would call me and say, "Thanks for calling, but we have already found somebody else." You know they were afraid of us, because of what happened when the first Albanians came. They think that we are all criminals, that we all steal, and therefore they are scared.

Together with Albanian workers, another im/migrant group that struggles to gain access into home eldercare assistance is African women. Here too not all African women have the same experience and once again certain nationalities are considered more *ideal* than others. For example, a study conducted in 2003 by the Italian National Social Security Institute (INPS) suggests that Ethiopian and Somali women are among the most favored groups for home eldercare assistance (INPS, 2003). Nevertheless during my participant observation at Tierra I witnessed a great amount of discrimination against African women in general. When an employer would call with a request for a domestic worker or a home eldercare assistant, the common practice for the mediator was to introduce three women from different nationalities. In all cases women from African backgrounds were the last resort and hardly ever got the job, and when they did, it was always for the most demanding live-in positions and the lowest wages. Sister Ortensia, the nun in charge of mediation between employers and employees at Benevolentia, observed similar patterns:

> There is a lot of discrimination linked to nationality, this year in particular because the market is saturated, but in general after 9/11 nobody wants to hire women from Morocco, not to mention African women. The color of the skin, it's still a huge issue. Therefore, in the end, they are the ones who take on the most difficult jobs, the ones with the least amount of freedom. And they take them only because they are desperate.

Discrimination related to skin color is expressed particularly by the elders, who still reflect colonial notions of difference. Italian elders having grown up during the brief Italian colonial experience[8] and in a country that was characterized more by outward migration than an internal one have more difficulties adapting to a diverse population. Although Italian elders are, unfortunately, often the source of the most offensive racist remarks, they are not the only ones to discriminate. Employers of all ages do as well and for this reason Carolina Cardenas (1998, p. 5) points out, "the Africans are the most difficult ones to place."

Race and nationality, however, are not the only elements of discrimination. As sister Ortensia points out, religion plays a great part too. Families prefer to hire women with a similar set of beliefs and practices that will not challenge those of the elders and their families. The distrust for people of different religions is heightened when connected with race, and therefore African Muslim women have a difficult time finding employers that respect their culture, their religion, and their religious practices. These difficulties often oblige these workers to remain locked in very demanding positions even when they would like to move on. Rahxma, a Somali woman who has worked as a live-in home eldercare assistant for the past 8 years with the same family, explains:

> If it was up to me I would change everything about this job, I would try to find something more interesting or at least work only half a day. But I have never said these things to the family I work for, not because I'm afraid, but because I'm used to working here, and above all because they respect different cultures, they respect my food, my way of cooking. They

> never ask me to buy things that I cannot touch according to my religion. They never asked me to buy wine, ham or pork. I can pray here, practice my religion. That's why I like to work here. It's not easy to find people who respect one's culture.

In addition to gender, race/ethnicity, nationality, and religion, other elements of discrimination in the construction and creation of hierarchies of labor are age and family status because home eldercare assistants, aside from being unskilled, cheap, and prone to care, also need to be constantly available and not distracted by personal lives, families, or other obligations.

The women interviewed for this study ranged from 19 to 58 years old, although the majority of them were in their late 30s. There are many reasons why women working as home eldercare assistants tend to be older. One is that young women usually work as home eldercare assistants only to gain entry into the labor market, but move away from the job as soon as they can, whereas women in their 30s and early 40s seem to linger longer in this profession, ultimately either becoming unable or unwilling to change occupations. As other scholars have noted, the passage of time in domestic and care work is often accompanied by a lowering of expectations and career ambitions (Kaufman, 2000). The relatively higher age of the women in home eldercare assistance, however, is also due to practices implemented by mediators in the three different organizations I observed. All three of them stated clearly that young women are not appropriate for eldercare and they actively discourage them from seeking these positions both for their own good and to offer employers more reliable employees. Mediators believe that younger women, due mostly to biological needs, are not the best match for this job. All the mediators suggested that older women are better at home eldercare assistance because of their greater patience, their ability to listen more carefully, and their lower expectations overall. In some cases, the employers themselves request women of specific ages. Sister Ortensia clarifies:

> Often employers themselves ask for a specific age, but for the elderly males we are the ones who choose to provide older women because there is always the risk of sexual abuse. It is a fine line and often the sons and daughters themselves that tell us, "my father is 85 years old but he is still sexually active" and therefore it's up to us to send somebody older, who at least would know how to put him in his place.

Inappropriate touching, molestation, and various degrees of sexual offers were a common thread in the interviews with im/migrant women and the cultural mediators, particularly when elderly males were involved. Nevertheless, the cultural mediators had no real solution for it, other than suggesting older women who were, in their opinion, potentially less attractive and more experienced in dealing with this kind of situation, which, in turn, shows an acceptance and normalization of the inappropriate behavior and enforces inequality between those offering care and those being cared for.

During my participant observation at Tierra, I watched Pilar, the Peruvian mediator, gently steering young women away from home eldercare assistance and redirecting them toward either domestic or factory jobs. The only young women who were directed toward home eldercare assistance were former sex workers who were in need of shelter and of a new job. At the same time, however, women who were perceived to be too old were steered away from live-in work. When Corina, a 59-year-old Peruvian woman came to the Tierra to look for work, Pilar kindly explained to her that she was too old to work, particularly at night.

Therefore, the ideal home eldercare workers are women whose age falls within a range from late 30s to mid-50s, the age in which women, particularly the traditional ones so desired by Italian employers, typically start a family and are raising children or caring for grandchildren. The ideal home eldercare assistant, according to Italian employers, has to be unencumbered by familial attachments. As mentioned at the beginning of this chapter one of the characteristics of the ideal home eldercare assistant is her ability to become, at least during the work relationship, a fictional member of the elders' families. To be able to fit that role the ideal employee needs to have the desire or the need to become part of the elders' families, and for this reason single women or women who have left their families behind are favored over those who have husbands and/or children with them. As Giulia's quote in the previous section indicates, children are seen as the greatest problem because their needs may endanger the quality and the amount of care provided to the elder. This concern was reiterated by Maurizia:

> When Irina asked me to hire her, she didn't have anybody, and she kept saying, "Take me, take me, I don't need to rest on the weekend; I can work all the time." So I did and at the beginning she was always with us, because she didn't have anybody, so on the weekend we would go to the country house all together with her, my mom, my brother and my daughter. In those months Irina really became one of the family.... Now that she brought her daughters in from Moldavia she no longer wants to spend the weekend with us; she wants her free time to be with her daughters.... I understand ... but I also need her to care for my mother who no longer wants anybody else.

Because of the specific requests made by the employers, mediators actively discourage women with families to take live-in jobs, and also, but to a lesser extent, to accept live-out ones, trying to redirect them to hourly domestic work. It is not by chance that out of 35 im/migrant women interviewed for this project 12 had no children, 4 had grown up offspring, and 5 left their children in their country of origin.

The preference for single women or women without children and/or a husband indicates, in general, that home eldercare assistance, like domestic and care work, encourages the migration of single women or women without their families and consequently of transnational motherhood (Hondagenu-Sotelo, 2001; Parreñas, 2001). However, it is important to note that there are exceptions to the rule. In fact, it is not uncommon for women who are already working to find ways to send for their children. As seen in Chapters 5 and 6, families that come to trust their employees will do everything to make sure that the employee will not leave them and that includes accommodating their immediate families and helping them secure permits of residence. Among the 13 women interviewed for this project who had to leave small children behind, eight were able to reunite with their children while working as home eldercare assistants.

CONCLUSIONS

In this chapter I outlined how im/migrant women coming to Italy from all corners of the world and from very different backgrounds in terms of class, education, and profession are transformed over time into the workers the growing market for long-term care requires. The home eldercare assistants needed by Italian families are not workers with specific skills and abilities, rather they are seen as "replacements" for the family caregivers. As such they cannot be themselves—who they really are in terms of social background, education, or class; rather they have to take on a persona designed for them by Italian society at large. This persona, who in order to satisfy the needs of employers has to reenact idealized notions of womanhood, gender, care, and culture, is extremely important because she allows for the recreation of a *fictional extended family* functional not only to Italian families but to the welfare state as well, which is dependent on these care arrangements. In this chapter I have described how the transformation of im/migrant women into home eldercare assistants happens at different levels: at the global level through the process of migration, and at the local level through the constant struggle to gain legal status in the country of arrival, and in the encounter with the actual employers. Through this process im/migrant women from different social, cultural, and class backgrounds are first stripped of their individual identity and become an undifferentiated group, that of im/migrant women in need of work. This first transformation allows for a second one, enforced by employers, in which im/migrant women are then transformed into the ideal workers needed by Italian families according to idealized hierarchies of race/ethnicity, religion, age, familial status, and more.

ACKNOWLEDGMENTS

Material in Chapter 5 is adapted from Francesca Degiuli, "Labouring Lives: The Making of Home Eldercare Assistants in Italy." In *Modern Italy*, 16(3), 2011, 345–361, Taylor and Francis Group.

NOTES

1 The only private structures that are attempting to obtain a foothold in this market are temporary agencies, but it is a relatively new phenomenon not fully developed.

2 Traditional according to the "ideology of the private sphere," the Victorian notion according to which women are better suited to the private sphere than the public one, a notion clearly expressed by the king, in Tennyson's *The Princess*:

> Man for the field and woman for the hearth:
> Man for the sword and for the needle she:
> Man with the head and woman with the heart:
> Man to command and woman to obey.

In this understanding women are seen according to maternalistic culture whereby women are 'naturally' prone to care.

3 The quote is taken from Pojman (2006, p. 6).

4 C. Ranci. Il welfare sommerso delle badanti. www.lavoce.it. The article appeared on December 2, 2002.

5 This notion was once again reiterated in 2011 when I re-interviewed Pilar. In the new interview she stated that "The elders complain a lot about Eastern European women. They think that those women do not have a culture of care, for them caring for an elder is like any other job."

6 For more discussion on the distinction between spiritual and menial work in home care and its gendered and racialized implications see Roberts, D. (1997). Spiritual and menial housework. *Yale Journal of Law and Feminism*, 9(1), 51–80.

7 It is interesting to note that of the two employers who most vehemently complained about employees forgetting who the real *woman of the house* was and of overstepping their boundaries, one was employing a Moldavian woman and the other a Romanian one. I never heard of similar complaints when the workers involved were women of color.

8 Some of these elders also fought in East Africa during World War II to defend the colonies of Somalia, Eritrea, and Ethiopia and their thinking is still deeply influenced by imperialist notions of power and superiority.

6

SKILLING THE UNSKILLED

THE MULTIPLE DIMENSIONS OF ELDERCARE

One morning, a few days after my family and I arrived in Turin, Italy, while I was still exploring our surroundings, I walked onto the balcony of our new apartment. I was taken there by a sound, a strange, continuous, haunting sound that I had been hearing intermittently day and night since our arrival. I walked outside and looking down I saw on the large terrace below a very old woman, extremely frail looking, who was sitting, hunched in a chair in the shadowy corner. Her face displayed no emotion and she seemed neither happy nor sad, but it was clear that the sound was coming from deep inside her. After a few minutes of standing there watching, an energetic looking woman with dark, short hair walked outside, took a chair, and sat next to the old woman. She started to talk to her in a sweet, friendly voice, a bit like one would do to calm down an agitated child, all the while caressing her hand. The younger woman spoke Italian fairly well, with only a hint of an Eastern European accent, and said "Nonna, why can't you calm down, what is bothering you, why can't you find some peace for you. . . and for me?" The older woman did not look like she was really listening, but her expression was beginning to change; there was a glint of understanding in her face, as if all of a sudden she was aware of no longer being alone. However, the lament did not stop. The younger woman then got closer to the old lady and hugged her tight, while beginning to sing a song—nothing I could understand, but her voice was very soft and sweet . . . it was an instant but I saw the older woman almost break into a smile as when one wakes up from a pleasant dream and for a short amount of time the lament did stop . . . and the silence felt almost overwhelming. The women and I were suspended in that silence for a little while, but it did not last. In what seemed less than a minute the older woman's face resumed her emotionless stare and the sound, that terrible sound started again (Turin, Fieldnotes, March 2004).

In the previous chapter I illustrated, among other things, what employers look for when selecting a home eldercare assistant and how they construct the ideal employee. Through this process employers also construct the job: they define it, they provide boundaries for it, and they attach a value to it. In the interviews employers describe the job, for the most part, as an extension of unpaid domestic work, an unskilled job that does not require particular abilities except those bestowed upon the workers by gender: sweetness, kindness, patience, and a certain upbringing usually associated with being a girl—being able to clean, organize, and manage a household, and most importantly being able to express some level of care and emotional empathy. This understanding of home eldercare assistance as an offshoot of domestic work goes well beyond the employers and is often supported by scholars, governmental institutions, media, and other social actors to the point that it can be difficult to obtain hard numbers differentiating between the two. Such a conflation is not necessarily arbitrary. Rather, it is born from the fact that the boundaries between the two occupations are often blurred. In this chapter, however, I argue that domestic work and home eldercare assistance are two different jobs with different goals, requiring a different set of skills and a different level of emotional involvement, but that im/migrant women often end up doing both due to our societal difficulties in attributing appropriate monetary value and recognition to what caring for the elders entails.[1]

To show the complexity of home eldercare assistance—how it differs from domestic work, and the many skills that it actually involves—in this chapter I provide a thorough description of what lies behind the simple label of *home eldercare assistant* by relying on the narratives of the im/migrant women who do this job. In addition, I also explore how very diverse the same job may be depending on the number of hours worked, the different living arrangements, and the physical and mental conditions of the elders in order to provide suggestions on how to improve both the working conditions of the immigrant workers and the well-being of the elders in their care.

THE JOB

The simple label "home eldercare work" encompasses a variety of work situations, yet suggests a job more homogeneous than the occupation actually is. To better understand the requirements of this occupation it is important to define what the label actually means. The first division runs between *live-in* eldercare work, which requires cohabiting with the elders 24 hours a day, usually for a minimum of 5 to a maximum of 7 days a week, and *live-out* eldercare work, which is usually defined by a shift of 8 hours a day 5 days a week. The other distinction is related to the physical and mental conditions of the elders. Some care workers tend to non-self-sufficient elders with various kinds of physical or mental disabilities ranging from Alzheimer's disease and Parkinson's disease to complete paralysis, whereas others simply provide companionship to frail elders, who, although self-sufficient, do not feel safe left alone. These different jobs generate different relationships, needs, and conflicts, but also share many similarities.

WAKING UP . . .

Viviana, a Peruvian in her early 40s caring for Lidia, 84 years old affected by Alzheimer's disease, explains:

> Yes, my day starts every day around 6 a.m., sometimes a bit earlier. At that time I usually wanted to keep sleeping but I couldn't because Lidia wanted her breakfast. The problem was that she didn't want the breakfast I could prepare for her. No, no, she wanted it from the neighborhood coffee shop. She wanted a latte and a croissant every morning, otherwise she wouldn't eat. So every morning from 6:00-7:15, the time the coffee shop would actually open, I had to find ways to entertain her, talk to her, cajole her into being quiet. When the clock would hit 7:15, I would run out of the house making sure to lock the door, otherwise she would escape, and hurry to the store to get her breakfast. At the coffee shop they already knew me, and as soon as they would see me they would prepare the latte. They knew that I was in a rush because if it took me too long to go back Lidia would begin to act crazy. She would scream, kick the door, and in order to get back into the house I had to calm her down and convince her that I wasn't a burglar but that it was me, Viviana, with her breakfast. After she had breakfast she would calm down and would go back to sleep, usually until 11:30 a.m. . . At that point, however, I was wide awake and I would begin to do my daily chores.

Viviana outlines how her workday begins as soon as she opens her eyes and it is immediately defined by the needs of the elder in her care. For most live-in workers the job begins right away, without the possibility of a personal daily routine: drinking a coffee, having breakfast, or showering. As soon as they open their eyes they have to become instantly available to the need of the elders, and in some cases, as Viviana explains, being present is not enough, rather it requires the enactment of multiple strategies to keep the elder calm, safe, and satisfied.

For live-out home eldercare assistants, instead, the workday is usually less hectic and it begins only when they walk into the house and the elders wake up. Afina, a Romanian woman in her early 40s caring for an elderly couple, tells quite a different story:

> The morning for us starts when Nora, the wife, wakes up, looks at me and says "oh dear, you're here." She is usually so happy to see me . . . I mean, it wasn't like that at the beginning. I had to win her trust, but now when she sees me, she knows that it is going to be a good day for her. After that I go to the kitchen and prepare the coffee. Antuan, the husband, joins me. We sit down and chat, drinking our coffee.

Breakfast is when the mood for the day is generally set, which is why it is very important for the home eldercare assistants to make sure that the elders start the day in a good mood. Breakfast, or soon after, is also the time when medications are administered and the medical needs of the elders such as cleaning bedsores, starting infusions, or giving injections are tended to. Notwithstanding the lack of formal training, most home eldercare assistants, along with physical and mental care, also perform some basic nursing skills,[2] with employers usually providing them with the medications and a timetable of when they need to be administered. More complex training, such as learning how to start and stop infusions or to do injections are sometimes provided unofficially by the Integrated Home Care Assistance's nurses who visit once a week or once every 15 days.[3] After breakfast the morning routine continues and usually involves sharing the most intimate aspects of everyday life with the elders. Luz, a 40-year-old Filipina, had to train Olga in a new bathroom routine:

> Right after breakfast is the time when I make sure that Grandma didn't make any mess because she has intestinal problems. The first two years I slept in the same room with her because she needed to talk, and she would talk all night, then she stopped, and I moved to my own room. . . [During that time] I didn't sleep for eight months in order to teach her how to go to the bathroom and now we finally developed a routine. Every morning after breakfast we go to the bathroom, I put on gloves and manually stimulate her anus. She suffers from severe constipation and at times I actually have to grab her poop with my hands. We even have a special language for it. We call the poop "princess." After that we shower, and then I brush her teeth, comb her hair, put on some make-up. We also choose the dress that she wants to wear for the day.

As Luz points out, home eldercare assistance involves a level of intimacy and closeness between the workers and the elders that is rarely, if ever, present in domestic work. The most intimate elements of the elders' bodies and lives become the territory that home eldercare assistants need to defend, protect, care for, and when possible, heal. This requires many skills. They need to gain trust, they need to show respect for the aging body and its needs, and they need to understand the difficulties inherent in accepting the aging process. In exchange, they are able to exert some level of power over the elderly bodies: they make decisions for them, they choose appropriate strategies, and they devise specific routines. Afrodita, a 38-year-old Albanian woman, adds:

> Some of my friends ask me, "Afrodita, how can you do that job? Aside from being hard work, you also have to change diapers. . ." and I always answer "Excuse me, but what about nurses in the hospitals? They do the same thing right? You put on gloves, clean, wash and dry up and it's all fine, no?"

Both Luz and Afrodita's words show that home eldercare assistants see themselves more as nurses than domestic workers. Their job, based on their own understanding of it, is to make sure that the body and the mind of the elders are taken care of first. Once the elder is clean and dressed for the day, and the medications have been administered, the rest of the morning is usually spent cleaning the house and buying groceries.

As mentioned in the introduction, domestic work remains an integral part of the job. Although most of the women are hired as eldercare assistants and not as maids, the notion that they will keep both the house and the elder clean is often an unspoken part of the agreement. If the worker does not immediately comply, the families tend to mention it in the first few weeks of work as Elvire, a 33-year-old woman from the Ivory Coast, recalls:

> It's always like that when they hire you. They ask you to do only certain things, for example just to look after grandma, make sure that she is clean and feed her. After a week they also ask you to clean the house and buy groceries. It never ends.

The lack of a written contract, the vulnerable position of most of these workers, and the vague job description allow employers to constantly reframe the terms of the work relationship. The workers, afraid to lose their jobs, their wages, and potentially their residence permits,[4] often comply without saying anything. However, what seems to hurt the workers most is the inability of the employers—the family—to understand that the *time of care* is very different from the *time of production* and that care work requires very different skills from domestic work. Elvire points out:

> The worst part of these jobs is not the elders or their needs. It's the family. They tend to disrespect you because they think that you're not really

> working, not really earning your money. It doesn't matter that you are locked inside the house with the elder 24 hours a day for five or seven days a week. They want to see you doing something all the time. That is why they keep giving you stuff to do. They don't understand that care work is not necessarily about being active all the time, but consists above all in being patient, listening, and trying to understand the elders' needs.

A similar concern is expressed by Madeline:

> I believe the elders have a lot of dignity, even if they are covered in poop, because when you wash them they are themselves again. Dignity goes beyond the human body. The daughters, the sons that hire us, they don't see all the care we have for their elders. They examine us on small things, unable to see that what matters is how we make their elder feel. They are not able to see or evaluate the relationship that we are able to create with the elder.

Time of care and *time of production*, as most of the home eldercare assistants emphasize, are very different. The first, time of care, is a time that in most postindustrial societies has completely lost value. It is a time that does not require constant measurable outputs, but one geared to create a sense of well-being for the person cared for. It is a time that may involve less cleaning and more listening, less cooking and more singing, less ironing and more laughing. Time of production, instead, is concerned with productivity—with the constant output of tangible services. Eldercare work, according to the women who do it, requires both, but for the job to be effective, the former has to be privileged over the latter. The families, while being well aware of the value of both "times," cannot control and regulate the time of care, cannot quantify its cost, and therefore tend to exert their control through the time of production. The description of the daily routines, although hinting at it, does not reveal in its real intensity the amount of emotional labor that is performed in these jobs. Luminita, a 51-year-old Romanian woman, describes this:

> With [the elders] one needs to be patient. Sometimes they scold you, then they want to kiss you, and then they ask you to leave again. One never knows what they really need. I do everything I can for them: I sing, I dance . . . I try to entertain them.

Aside from performing practical tasks, what most of these women do in these jobs is to give the elders a part of themselves, of their desire to be alive, of their personal histories, of their future, of their dreams. These women share with the elders a large part of their private selves and, sometimes, even their children. But although doing all this in exchange for wages, the women do not consider this aspect of their occupation as exploitative (Hochschild, 2003). On the contrary, for the most part, they consider performing this *love work* a redeeming aspect of the job, what makes it worthy and irreplaceable. Lais, a Brazilian woman in her mid 30s, explains:

> When I began to do this job years ago it felt as if I had found myself, as if I had always done it and I was good at it. I like this job because it rewards me, every time I walk into their house [the elder couple she works for] and notice that they are happy to see me, I become happy too. Aside from the salary, which obviously I need, these things give me satisfaction. Working with the elders is satisfying because no matter how little you give them, they enjoy it, because they feel lonely and instead I like to chat and laugh. I keep them company. Even when I'm tired at the end of the day, to see them happy because of my presence gives me a jolt of energy.

The domestic chores are usually followed by morning errands; the daily groceries, in fact, are an important aspect of Italian everyday life, particularly for the older generations who are used to buying them daily in the neighborhood shops or street markets. Afina explains:

> While we drink the coffee in the morning, Antuan and I write down the list of the things that they want to eat for the day. Antuan gives me the money and I go out. I buy everything fresh everyday. They eat well, they eat good things, and I hope that they will always have enough money to eat like this, but at the moment they are well, really well.

The act of going out to buy groceries fulfills more than simply the need to provide food. It allows the elders to remain in contact with the larger society; therefore, when they are still able to walk they often accompany the home eldercare assistants in these errands. Veronica, a 47-year-old Peruvian woman, remembers how much they enjoyed these walks before the elderly lady of the couple she was looking after became too ill:

> After breakfast Giovanni, Maria, and I would walk to the street market. That was when both were still healthy. They loved the daily routine, the stop at the bakery, sometimes at the butcher, to look at the fresh vegetables and fruit at the street market. Mostly they liked being out and being recognized. They knew everybody in the neighborhood and everybody would salute them. Once Maria got sick we had to let go of our daily walks.

The daily errands are also an important time for the majority of live-in workers because errands allow them to leave the house, break the monotony of the twosome relationship with the elders, reenter the reality of the external world, and establish friendly relations in the neighborhood; they also learn about Italian culture, something that the elders are very attached to. Gladys, a Peruvian woman in her mid 50s, learned how to cook Italian dishes from an Italian woman selling vegetables at the street market:

> My first job as an elder assistant was with a blind lady and I had to do everything for her, but I didn't know where to start because in my country I had a girl who would do the domestic work for me and another woman that would cook for us. I didn't have any experience in domestic work. I was not able to cook and even worse I was working for a blind lady who wasn't able to teach me anything. I learned how to cook from the lady where I would buy fresh produce at the street market. She was kind and explained how to cook the things that I was buying.

For some live-in workers, however, even that short amount of freedom is accompanied by apprehension because of the elder's physical and mental conditions and the worker's own sense of responsibility. Luz says:

> I don't leave Olga for more than thirty minutes. That is the amount of time I allow myself to buy groceries. I can't leave her alone longer than that because in the past she attempted suicide. She did it while I was already working for her. I became very ill after that, I had to go to the hospital, so my conscience troubles me if I leave her longer than that.

After the groceries are done, it is usually time for the domestic chores. Afrodita, who used to work as a live-in eldercare assistant, together with her 3-year-old son, describes her routine as follows:

> Once back home, after I left my child in day care I would begin to clean the house while Gina was still in bed. She was such a lazy one (laughs). Every day I would dust, sweep and mop all the floors, clean the bathroom, the kitchen, do the laundry, and iron all of our clothes. It was only a two-bedroom apartment, but I tell you, it was enough to keep me busy.

LUNCHTIME

Lunchtime and the activities involved in it such as cooking and sharing meals are also important parts of the daily routine. For some women the time spent preparing the meal is a pleasant moment in the day because it helps them to bond with the elders and allows them to learn new recipes and different ways of cooking. For others, instead, the meals are a difficult time because they often bring to the fore cultural differences that are frequently disrespected by the Italian elders. Carmen, 28, a woman from Ecuador explains:

> When I began to work for this lady, I didn't know how to cook Italian food, and it was a big deal because she was Sicilian and food was really important to her. She would get angry about it. I had to learn to cook all her favorite dishes and that was fine, I like to cook. . . . The main problem was that she didn't let me buy nor cook the food I liked. And it was hard because, aside from missing my family and my son, I wasn't even able to eat the food I was used to. It was as if I had lost another part of myself.

After preparing lunch, home eldercare assistants are often asked to share the meal with the elders. Sharing the meals is important for them and the task is often perceived by the workers as part of their job requirements. Afrodita remembers:

> She would constantly ask me "Afrodita, please sit down, eat with me," and I always felt that I had to do it even if I didn't feel like eating. It was important for her to share the meals with me; she didn't like to eat alone. If I didn't do it she would get mad at me, tell me that I offended her and would be unbearable all day.

While for some elders this activity is considered a convivial gesture and an attempt to break the barriers between employers and employees, for others it becomes a way to control and determine what the employee can eat and when. Workers, particularly those in their first job, often complained of not being fed enough, or having to eat food that did not belong to their culture or that they simply did not like. Sharing meals for some elders means that they no longer consider the worker simply a "worker" but also a member of the family. Therefore, they try to maintain this ritual even when the job no longer requires it. Lucha, a 51-year-old Peruvian woman, recounts:

> I worked for the same family for seven years, mostly to take care of the wife, but she passed away. The husband keeps reducing my hours because he feels that he doesn't need me as much, but the thing I really don't like is the fact that he keeps insisting that we eat together at lunch, but he doesn't pay me for that time and I don't think it's right. . . .

This quote emphasizes how the boundaries between work and daily life are often blurred in these work relations and how some employers tend to misunderstand the relationship that links them to the worker. In this case the employer does not understand that Lucha perceives the shared meal as a part of her job and not as a convivial activity or as a special tie. Once again the quote highlights the difficulties that employers have in seeing companionship, in this case the sharing of a meal, as something that should be considered work and as such properly paid.

THE AFTERNOON

The early afternoon is usually a time during which the daily activities slow down. After a busy morning, the majority of the elders need time to rest: some watch TV, some nap, and some talk on the phone with friend and relatives. This is the time when live-in workers usually take advantage of their daily time off. For most of them it simply involves going to their rooms to read a newspaper, to call home, to take care of themselves, or to go out for a walk. The time off is when the different coping strategies to combat the difficulties of the job, the sense of loneliness, and the hope for improvement are displayed. Some women use this time to call their friends or family on the phone in order to feel less lonely. They talk with their children, husbands, and relatives or call other women doing the same job to vent about difficult days, elders, or employers in general. Others use this time to improve their education, learn new skills, or apply for more satisfactory jobs. Finally, for a few others it means being able to go to their own home. Some of the workers choose to maintain a room or an apartment shared with others even when working full-time. This decision is often considered a survival strategy and even if it is a difficult choice because of the huge toll it has on their wages and consequently on their remittances, the funds spent on a separate space is considered money well spent.

RESUMING THE WORK

Once the resting time is over for both the elders and the workers the workday resumes and the tasks are very similar to the ones performed in the morning. The disabled elders need to be changed and cleaned again, and a second round of medication often needs to be administered. Afina, for example, needs to be back at work exactly at 3:45 because that is the time when Nora usually needs to go to the bathroom and without Afina, Nora would not be able to do it:

> I need to be there precisely at that time because she is used to her routine. I can't be late because if something happens I would feel terrible, plus it's my job. I have to be there when she needs me.

Once the elders, after the laborious care of the workers, are again ready to resume their daily routine, the late afternoon is usually spent in social activities. The most disabled elders who cannot go out are often condemned to be passive spectators, but even for them the workers try to find some solution in order to let the elders participate in social life. Afrodita mentions:

> In the afternoon I would always make sure to push grandma to make an effort and move from the bed to the wheelchair. She wasn't able to go out anymore but at least on the chair I was able to carry her out on the balcony. I would then leave her there, at least for an hour, so that she could look at people, and see what was going on in the neighborhood.

For those elders less physically ill or affected only by mental disorders, but still able to move on their own, the afternoon can be the peak of the day, the time in which the elders can fulfill their need for social contact. It usually involves walking around the neighborhood, going for coffee or tea at the neighborhood cafe, or, for some, going to church. It is an important part in the elders' day and it is lived as a very special moment. Viviana explains:

> When Lidia would wake up after her afternoon nap, she had to go out, so I would once again take her to the bathroom, clean her up, comb her hair, put make up on, I mean I would take on so many roles: the hairdresser, the esthetician, I would do everything, everything, because I really took good care of her. We would put on a dress, not the same one that she was wearing in the morning, but a new one and then we were ready to go out. At that point it was almost four in the afternoon, and we would go say hi to all the people who she knew, because you have to keep in mind that in the neighborhood everybody knew her, and she was so happy, then when she would get bored with one person we would move to the next, and she would chat a little more, and that routine was really good for her, it used to make her feel good.

Viviana's account emphasizes two important points. The first point is that during a typical day home eldercare assistants constantly shift among different roles: from assistant to fictive family member, from nurse to hairstylist, from cook to chaperon. All with one goal in mind, that of making the elder feeling cared for, nurtured, and still important in people's lives. This constant shifting shows that the job is anything but unskilled. On the contrary, it requires many different sets of skills that may vary from situation to situation. The second point is the importance of social interaction for the elders. As already mentioned in the morning section, interaction with a larger society is a very important aspect of eldercare and home eldercare assistants are central in maintaining these connections, showing that fellowship is as essential to eldercare as many of the other more practical tasks. Caring for the elders, in fact, does not simply mean making sure that they are comfortable, clean, and well fed, it also entails helping them to maintain social relationships and a place in the larger society.

Although taking the elder for a walk in a public square or park or to get a coffee at the neighborhood bar may seem like nonessential work, not "real work," it actually fulfills a very important function in the lives of the elderly and it is a crucial part of the caring process. Studies show that the elders who are involved in some form of social interaction maintain better physical and mental health (among others Alden, 2011; Murray & Crummet, 2010; Reichstadt, Sengupta, Depp, Palinkas, & Jeste, 2010; Unger, Ander Johnson, & Marks, 1997).

EARLY EVENING

Six thirty or seven is usually the time when the workday ends for most of the live-out workers. It is the moment in the day when family members return home from work or when other workers take on the night shift. Most live-out workers enjoy this time of the day, not only because it is the end of work duties, but, above all, because it allows them to "emotionally close the door on the job" as Maria, a 38-year-old Peruvian woman puts it, and, at the same time, to resume their personal lives. Aline, a Brazilian worker in her mid 30s explains:

> To go to work and come back home I take the train. It is usually a thirty-minute ride. I love that time because it allows me to remove myself from the elder's life and to come back to mine. I enjoy that separation. . . . What is difficult with these jobs is the constant sharing. . . the forced cohabitation. Now that I have a life of my own, a life separate from the job, it is completely different. The job becomes a job like any other; I even like it.

However, for the majority of elders' assistants the job does not end here but continues, in some cases, late into the night. The evening routine is similar to the lunch one. When the physical conditions allow for it the elders usually participate in the preparation of the meal and, if feeling well enough, also in sharing the meal with the rest of their own or their adopted families. Irina, clarifies:

> The evening meal is usually a more crowded and louder meal because my daughters are home from school, my husband, who lives downstairs, is back from work and Anna and Laura [Sara's daughter and granddaughter] are, often, here too. If Sara feels well enough we enjoy eating all together so that she can participate a bit in everybody's lives.

Usually, though, the meals are shared only between the elders and their assistants. The respective families are absent for very different reasons. The workers' families have been left behind either in the country of origin or at their new home in Italy to allow the worker to do her job. The elders' families, instead, are absent for various reasons: some live in other cities, some believe that their lives are already difficult enough to manage without the burden of an ailing relative, and some have their own families to take care of, whereas others actually fear witnessing their parents decay and are unable to face it first hand. In all these cases the elders and the workers end up sharing their different solitude, one stemming from old age in industrial societies and the other from the need to provide remittances in a globalized economy.

EVENING/NIGHT

The time after dinner is dedicated, once again, to cleaning: first the kitchen and then, if the elder is disabled, the elder himself or herself. The evening is also a time when the eldercare assistants try to prepare the elders for the night, not only by tending to their physical needs but also by attempting to create a serene and calm atmosphere in which to take care of the spiritual needs of the elders: assuage their fears, dull their emotional pain, and relieve their loneliness. Luzviminda talks about what she and Olga do at this time of the day:

> Olga has Alzheimer's but she understands everything. For example, I don't let her watch the news because it agitates her. So in the evening if we don't go to church, I make her listen to "Radio Maria," a Catholic radio station, because I think that, even if she doesn't believe in God, listening to their programs helps her to relax. I often tell her: "Guga, your life may be almost over, but your duty as a human being is not over, you have to pray for other people."

Luzviminda's words draw attention to the fact that home eldercare assistants are not simply the hands of the employers, but they have a certain level of power not only in deciding how to handle the elders physically, but also emotionally and spiritually. In the case of home eldercare assistance, unlike other forms of domestic and care labor, the boundaries between spiritual and menial labor (Roberts, 1997) become more fluid and home eldercare assistants, in some cases, end up doing both.

Taking care of the elders' emotional needs at night is important not only for the elders who will then be able to have a restful sleep, but also for the assistants who otherwise will have to keep working well into the night. Viviana explains:

> Lidia couldn't sleep. Every night after watching TV, around 11:30 or 12:00 I would give her a sleeping pill and put her in bed. I would wish her a good night, turn off the light and leave the room. After only an hour though she would call me and would say "Viviana, please, turn on the light, I don't want to be in the dark." Then she wanted to tell me about her mother, her

> father, and many other things of her life and I would sit there and listen... Then around 3 or 4 a.m. she would fall asleep and I would do the same on my chair. She usually would sleep from 3:30, 4 am to 6, and at that time the breakfast routine would start all over again...

As can be seen from these descriptions, the workday for a live-in assistant can be never ending. Women such as Viviana, Rahxma, Luz, Afrodita, Elvire, and many others work 24 hours a day without boundaries either of space or time. Constantly being in the workplace also means that they are constantly available for the elders, day and night. Even if, in some cases, the work is not hard because the elders are in good physical condition and sleep through the night, the lack of freedom makes this job difficult to bear. Teresa, a 38-year-old woman from Ecuador who helps place im/migrant women in care jobs in her position at Benevolentia, explains:

> I've done a number of jobs since I came here. I worked in a restaurant, I worked as a domestic, as chef-aid, as a manager in the same restaurant and in a factory. I worked with elders only twice, but it was the best job because if one is lucky it can even be relaxing, and one doesn't spend any money. Instead working in a factory is much more alienating. The real problem in working with the elders is the lack of freedom. The fact of not being able to go out was terrible. I honestly felt like a sparrow in a golden cage where one has everything for his or her well-being, but freedom. The job is all right if the elder is in relatively good shape and you can go out together, otherwise it becomes suffocating.

Rahxma, who has worked as a live-in assistant for 8 years, adds:

> I miss my freedom; I have been doing this job for eight years. I lived with this lady since I was 24 and I miss my life. There are so many things that I would like to do but I can't.... How can I put it? I dislike 80% of this job simply because of the lack of freedom. There is nothing about this job that bothers me: I like the woman I work for, I like doing things for her but I want a life of my own, I want to be able to leave work and go home, see my friends, leave all this behind.

Not all women have such a positive description of their living arrangements or of their employers, but they agree on how difficult it is to be locked in all day. The lack of freedom, while being the predominant disadvantage of live-in work, is not the only one. The inability to leave the job behind at the end of the day is another aspect that makes it difficult to endure. Physical exhaustion is also a problem because, as we have seen throughout the chapter, live-in workers may be on call all the time. In addition to mental and physical exhaustion, home eldercare assistants also experience extreme loneliness. The social world of live-in workers often includes only the person they care for, and sometimes, but not always, the family of the elder and occasional interactions during the daily errands.

Other difficulties related to this job involve the inability of workers to control their own living conditions. Unlike domestic work and child care, elder care work is not relegated only to the upper and middle classes, and therefore elder care assistants may end up experiencing all sorts of living conditions. In most cases the apartments that the workers and the elders share are small and the two worlds end up constantly colliding. Elvire, for example, remembers that at her first job she had to share the same bed with the elder she was caring for because the apartment was so tiny that there was no other place where she could sleep. Forced cohabitation in small environments is difficult, even with a friend, but it can become almost unbearable with a perfect stranger whose habits differ greatly from your own. Work ends up filling every moment of these women's lives, leaving little or no space for anything else. Live-in im/migrant women, in a way, become hostage to their employers. In time most of these workers learn to defend their rights and their privacy, but it is a difficult process that first requires acquiring a certain proficiency with the language, and second a certain amount of bargaining power usually acquired by either becoming "irreplaceable" or by obtaining a residency permit. In any case, it is not by chance that as soon as it becomes feasible, im/migrant women workers try to move away from live-in work and go back to it only when in need of a place to stay or when they cannot find other employment.

For some, however, live-in work is not merely the best alternative among very limited options, but may become an active choice. Some women choose live-in work because they have short-term migratory projects and live-in jobs allow them to save as much money as possible and consequently to send larger remittances home. Others choose it because living-in provides temporary shelter in the nest of another family. Finally, there are women such as Luz who decide to make live-in eldercare work their profession. Here she outlines the different reasons that convinced her to keep doing this job:

> I did this job for 16 years. I worked as a live-in for the entire time and I assure you it's not easy. One needs to be very strong mentally. I like to work with the elders for three reasons: because I hate the cold and I don't want to be running all over town from one job to another, because I was a nurse obstetrician in the Philippines and I know what it means to take care of people. For us in the Philippines the elders are like precious artifacts in a museum. We need to take good care of them. I was used to taking care of my grandmother and I grew up valuing elders and, finally, because I like it, I call it a vocation. I can do this job even with my eyes closed.

Live-out eldercare work does not have the same negative connotation as live-in work. On the contrary, many consider the job as good as any other and one that can actually be very satisfactory from an emotional point of view. Afrodita explains:

> I like to help, I like to spend time with the elders . . . even if . . . I mean we all are unbearable when we don't feel well, when we have a headache we become obnoxious, therefore the elders too, poor souls, their bodies are breaking down, but in any case I like to work with them. Seriously, I really like the job, but certainly not 24 hours a day and with a kid on top of that as I did for 18 months. That never again, but eight hours a day, or half a day sure no problem, with all my heart.

However, even when confined to 8 hours a day, the job, for many im/migrant workers, often remains unsatisfactory because of the poor wages, the low social status attached to it, and the lack of social recognition.

CONCLUSIONS

The description of the daily routines of both live-in and live-out im/migrant women workers reveals that home eldercare assistance is a labor-intensive occupation both in terms of productive and emotional labor. The accounts also show that although home eldercare assistance is often described simply as an offshoot of domestic work, it actually is a different occupation that requires a different set of skills, goals, and priorities. During a typical 24-hour day home eldercare assistants perform a great number of practical tasks including cooking, cleaning, administering medications, cleaning wounds, helping the elders with the most intimate daily routines, keeping them mentally active, and allowing them to still take an active part in everyday life, while at the same time performing a great deal of emotional labor that ranges from the simple yet demanding need to always display appropriate body and facial expressions to devising complex tactics to keep the elders content, mentally active, and feeling part of the larger society. During their long workdays, home eldercare assistants, who are defined as unskilled workers, take on different roles, each requiring a different set of skills: from maid to chaperone, from nurse to hairstylist, and from cook to spiritual counselor, with each role addressing a different aspect of care.

The accounts of the im/migrant home eldercare assistants highlight different dimension of eldercare. The first dimension is that of body care: home eldercare assistants are responsible for maintaining the physical condition of the elderly body so that it is functional and comfortable through cleaning, bathing, feeding, and dressing, but also through embellishing it with makeup if that is part of the elder's routine and nurturing it with touch and massage. The elderly body, like the body of a child, needs to be handled gently, but it also needs to be treated with patience and kindness because it is a body that is slowing down and progressively losing its functions. It is a body that needs to be understood and respected even while losing all of its dignity.

The second dimension of eldercare is the emotional one. Home eldercare assistants sing, cajole, joke, dance, pray, dispel fears, comfort, connect, and sometimes make choices for the elders. Elderly patients are on a difficult journey, and as their bodies are shutting down, so are their minds. Even when they are not affected with Alzheimer's disease the elders forget things, feel vulnerable, and experience bouts of senile dementia that may make them angry, diffident, and downright intractable. As in the case of the body, the mind is slowing down and the process is often frustrating and painful for the elders and must be treated with compassion and understanding by the eldercare assistant.

A third important function of home eldercare involves helping the elders to maintain a connection with the outside world. Home eldercare assistants are crucial in keeping the elders connected to the larger society and helping them to maintain a presence in everyday life. By taking the elders for walks, buying groceries, and accompanying them to the public square, the church, or the neighborhood café, home eldercare assistants help the elders to remain engaged with the outside world and feel active and part of their communities.

Each dimension is connected to the others in a continuum of tangible and intangible tasks: home eldercare assistants need to clean the elders, brush them, dress them, and make them feel safe and comfortable, while at the same time showing a sense of deep respect for who the elders are and who they used to be. Home eldercare assistants have to cook and feed the elders while making sure that they respect the elders' culture, their habits, and their daily routines. The progressive loss that aging entails and the rage and despair associated with it can make elders experience mood swings and loss of words, so eldercare assistants must always be looking for ways to inject life, optimism, and happiness into bodies that often do not have any strength, both mental and physical, left in them. They have to deal with the complex turns of a mind symptomatic of senile dementia and the disappearing boundaries between reality and memory. All of these are tasks that may be summarized simply as *fellowship,* but that in reality are much harder and more complex than simply cleaning dishes, mopping floors, and buying groceries. Unlike domestic workers, home eldercare assistants are not relegated to simply performing menial tasks (Roberts, 1997); they are also in charge of the spiritual elements of caring for a human being. In the end, they are the ones who devise strategies, implement tactics, and design the best way to make the elderly comfortable.

Employers, however, still struggle in attributing a value to the invisible elements of care and often tend to push the workers to perform work that they can see and quantify, thus the conflation with domestic work and the constant tension between *time of care* and *time of production*[5]. In many countries of the world domestic workers still struggle to see their work and their rights properly recognized, but in some countries such as Italy they have been recognized as regular workers worthy of a national contract.[6] Home eldercare assistants are not quite there yet. Therefore

I argue that a full recognition of the value of care in all its dimensions is essential to designing a social pact that will protect both the increasing numbers of elders in need of care and the many workers who will be needed to care for them.

In addition, it is clear that although home eldercare assistants take pride in devising strategies and tactics to respond to the elders' needs they are not properly trained to do so. The lack of training may lead to haphazard solutions, and, at times, to abusive, albeit well-intentioned, behavior. While turning the home eldercare assistant job into a full profession may be difficult because it would raise the cost of labor, a publicly provided support line for home eldercare assistants would be extremely beneficial to both the workers and the elders. It would allow home eldercare assistants to obtain support from a number of professionals, including geriatric doctors, nurses, and social workers who could provide them with the help they need in facing complex pathologies ranging from Parkinson's disease to Alzheimer's disease, from senile dementia to type two diabetes, and more. It would also make the elders feel safer and more comfortable in knowing that they are being taken care of, albeit at a distance, from professionals trained in the care of geriatric patients.

Finally, the working conditions involved in these jobs should be somewhat legislated to prevent employers from abusing the workers and to maintain some level of equity among all im/migrant workers. Home eldercare assistance should be seen as a job different from domestic work and as such should be recognized and managed to accommodate these differences. Although other scholars have pointed out that working conditions for domestic and care workers vary greatly depending on the workers' relationship with the employers (live-in or live-out working arrangements) or on their relationship with the state (whether they have papers or not), I argue that an equally important variable in home eldercare assistance is the physical and mental condition of the elder being assisted. The amount of both productive and emotional labor increases greatly when the elders are completely disabled or when they are affected by complex pathologies such as Alzheimer's disease or Parkinson's disease. As represented in my interviews, some workers are on the job 24 hours a day for 5 or 7 days a week, whereas others work only a day or night shift. Some workers care for perfectly self-sufficient elders whereas others take care of those who are bedridden. Some simply need to provide companionship whereas others have to learn to deal with complex pathologies such as senile dementia or Parkinson's disease. These different elements have huge consequences for the daily experiences of the eldercare assistants and their ability to actively respond to the overwhelming demands of these jobs. Furthermore, the interviews reveal that even though, in general, workers prefer live-out jobs, and they will actively seek them as soon as they obtain residence permits, there are some cases in which they continue to prefer live-in arrangements independent of their im/migrant status. These exceptions include workers who have short-term migratory projects, have troubled relationships, are waiting to gain legal status, or conceive of the job as a vocation, as well as workers who, due to their race and religious beliefs, do not have easy access to other jobs or who, due to the great emotional attachment that these work relationships generate, tie their lives to those of the elders in their care. Proper legislation should take all these different elements into account and provide enough flexibility to allow for different kinds of services.

ACKNOWLEDGMENTS

Material in Chapter 6 is adapted from Francesca Degiuli, "A Job with No Boundaries: Home Eldercare Work in Italy." In *European Journal of Women's Studies*, 14(3), August 2007, 193–207, SAGE journals.

NOTES

1 This is applicable not only to Italy but also to the United States. While thanks to a new ruling passed by the Department of Labor starting from January 16th the majority of home care employees will be included in the Fair Labor Standard Act thereby gaining access to a minimum wage and to paid overtime, some will continue to remain excluded. Those are: "individual workers who are employed only by the person receiving services or that person's family or household and engaged primarily in fellowship and protection (providing company, visiting or engaging in hobbies) and care incidental to such activities," (http://www.dol.gov/whd/media/press/whdpressVB3.asp?pressdoc=national/20130917.xml)

2 Usually instructions regarding medications are provided by the employers whereas more complex training involving injections or infusions is often provided by the Integrated Home Care Assistance's nurses who visit once a week or once every 15 days.

3 When my mother was terminally ill with cancer, the nurses of the Home Care Integrated Program came over and trained both me and Dalisay, who at the time was caring for my mother during the day.

4 The permit-of-stay granted to im/migrant workers either through quotas or through amnesty lasts at most 2 years. After that workers need to renew it and to do that, among other requirements, they have to demonstrate that they are employed. For this reason even legal workers remain at the mercy of their employers. http://www.stranieriinitalia.it/italiano/page1/soggiorno.htm

5 Or, as in the case of the United States, the need to distinguish between productive tasks and the provision of fellowship.

6 According to historian Raffaella Sarti (2013) domestic workers were fully recognized in Italian labor legislation for the first time in 1958.

7

THE BONDS OF LABOR

"Everybody in the Filipino community talks about this story, everybody knows about it. Mari worked with this lady for six years. The lady lived in a big apartment all by herself and Mari would keep her company. They were always together, the old lady had a daughter, but she was not here, she had married and lived in Liguria (two hours away from Turin). Mari and the old lady were inseparable and Mari had a good life because the lady was in good shape, they went to visit the daughter at the seaside in the summer, they went to Church together, but one day the elderly lady fell and she broke her femur, after that she was not herself anymore. Mari was always at her side, helping her with everything, she was more than a daughter. This went on for a while but after eight months the lady died. Mari was very sad, also because she had to leave the apartment right away and she did not know where to go. A week after while she was staying with her aunt she received a phone call. It was the daughter of the old lady. You wouldn't believe it she called to tell Mari that the old lady had left her the apartment, the big apartment she had... Not to the daughter.... she left it to Mari, can you believe it? To Mari...." (Ligaya, conversation after the formal interview, March 2004)

Emotions, as seen in the previous chapter, are a central component of home eldercare assistance. The description of a typical 24-hour workday for both live-in and live-out home eldercare assistants reveals a job that creates a great deal of intimacy between the workers and the elders for whom they care. The constant sharing of space, meals, and daily intimate routines as well as the loneliness of both subjects involved in this work relationship help to generate a great deal of emotional attachment on both sides. These accounts reflect the findings of many care scholars according to whom paid care work differs from other market exchanges precisely because of the emotions that permeate the transaction (England, 2005). Feminist economist Nancy Folbre (2001), for example, described care work as a form of labor that is motivated, not simply by money, but also by the concern for the welfare of other people. Another economist, Susan Himmelweit (1999), has stated that the essence of care work itself defies its complete commoditization. Carework, in fact, entails both a personal and an emotional involvement of the worker, one that cannot be adequately captured, regulated, or monetized by the market in which it is bought and sold (Rodriguez, 2011, p. 265). Eldercare work, as other forms of carework, reflects the difficulties involved in managing the emergence of genuine emotions inside the confines of a work relationship that, in the Italian case, often involves three different actors: the im/migrant workers, the elders, and the family employers. The nature of these relationships varies a great deal because on the one hand it involves intimate interactions for extended periods of time between the home eldercare assistants and the elders for whom they care, and on the other hand it involves a less intimate and more formal relationship between the home eldercare assistants and the family members who hire them. In this chapter I explore what role emotions play in defining the boundaries of these triangular relationships of labor. In the process I argue that although emotional labor has largely been described in negative terms, it also provides an opportunity for agency (Ibarra, 2002; Rodriguez, 2011; Stacey, 2011). While it is clear that the relationship of power in home eldercare assistance tips in favor of the elders and their families, home eldercare assistants are able to use emotions and emotional attachments to elicit different kinds of help and support from their employers and to obtain some level of bargaining power that, in turn, allows them to improve their working or living conditions and/or their visa status.

CARING FOR A LIVING

Live-in jobs are, in many cases, the first step in im/migrant women's journey to Italy, and for a large number of them the jobs coincide with their first separation from their own family. Viviana explains:

> I like to work with the elders because they are in need, they rely on you, they make you feel useful, and most importantly they keep you busy, because an immigrant here, especially if alone without a family, if she is not busy she becomes depressed, she becomes sad, she begins to wonder about her kids: how are they doing, what are they up to, are they well or not. Instead if the elder keeps you busy it's not that hard. Plus it is easy to grow affectionate with them, because after the initial distrust, they fall in love with you and appreciate what you do for them, they really do.

This separation, combined with the inability to speak the language, the unfamiliarity with the new country, the long work hours, the lack of a private space, and the almost symbiotic relationship with the elder in their care, tends to create a strong emotional attachment toward the elders and their families. Aline remembers:

> The first two experiences I had as an eldercare assistant were very difficult because I used to get too attached to the person in my care. They were my first contact with a new reality, a new life, a new society. And because I didn't really speak Italian back then they were also my only connection with the rest of the world. Plus I didn't know anybody here and I missed my parents so it was easy to get attached to them, and they did treat me as a family member so in a way it was easy to do it, but then when the jobs ended it was so painful, so hard.

The emotional attachment that Aline mentions is a key point in these working relations because home eldercare work, unlike institutional and professional caring jobs, does not require a professional detachment and it is not closely defined by management (Lopez, 2006). It is also different from the home care provided by American care workers who engage directly with the elders in a private space (Stacey, 2011). In the Italian case families are involved even when not directly present and they actively encourage emotional involvement considering it an essential aspect of the job. As mentioned in Chapter 4, when families decide to hire a home eldercare assistant they are not looking for a trained professional, even when the elders may need it, rather they seek a substitute for themselves. What they are looking for, ideally, is someone possibly even better then themselves: somebody more patient, more available, and less distracted by other daily entanglements. They are not necessarily looking for someone "socially dead," as Anderson (2000) suggested, but for somebody whose life is temporarily on hold. And im/migrant women who have just entered the country provide just that: people whose prior skills and knowledge are no longer recognized, whose inability to speak the language isolates them from the rest of society, and whose loneliness and desire for affection can be matched only by the elders for whom they care. The quote, however, also emphasizes that these feelings and these attachments, although strong, are not supposed to last. When the relationship of labor ends, in many cases, so should the emotional bond. Aline's quote emphasizes the constant tension between home/work, insider/outsider, and public/private that home eldercare assistants have to negotiate on a daily basis. Home eldercare assistants have, on one hand, to perform specific tasks required by the family caregivers/employers that provide them with wages and, on the other hand, they do so in an environment that they struggle to consider a workplace and through emotions and tasks that belong to the private space rather than to the public one (Hochschild, 1983; Huang & Yeoh, 2007; Steinberg & Figart, 1999). This tension is constantly present and is negotiated in different ways depending on the level of experience of the home eldercare assistant, the relationship with the family, and the bond with the elder.

CREATING A BOND

The relational nature of eldercare assistance requires a continuous and often reciprocal emotional connection with the elder (Parks, 2003; Stacey, 2011). For this reason, eldercare entails much more than simply physical labor, it also calls for the worker's entire being: her mind, her emotions, her past, her future, and her dreams. Throughout their workday and notwithstanding the kind of practical tasks they are accomplishing, home eldercare assistants need to be kind, patient, and friendly, and to do so they have to put their heart on the line. Afina explains:

> If you put your heart and your soul in this job, then you work well, but if you have a cold heart . . . for this job one needs a lot of patience . . . if you have a cold heart, you can't do this job because the elders are very needy.

The emotional bond is so central to this job that when a worker is not able to establish it the work relationship becomes unsustainable and needs to be terminated. Luminita, a Romanian worker in her late 30s, explains:

> This job is difficult because one works at home always in touch only with the person we care for and if that person has a bad temper the job becomes unbearable. I understand that sick people may be nervous but when the person you care for is always nervous, always upset and you can't communicate, it's better for both of us to look for somebody else.

According to the narratives of the workers as well as the employers interviewed for this project, what the elders need, together with physical care, is the presence of somebody who makes them feel safe, loved, respected, and, most importantly, still alive. They need somebody who they can trust with their aging bodies and minds, specifically somebody who will not take advantage or make fun of failing memories, weak and trembling bodies, and deeply wrinkled skin. Luz, a Filipina worker, clarifies:

> The elders need to know that there is somebody who loves them. I can't change them or change the fact that they are going to die. The only thing I can do is to share my life with them.

The structure of the job itself together with its location, the private home of the elder, encourages the development of strong emotional ties. During their day, and sometimes night, the elders and the workers spend a great deal of time together, often completely removed from the rest of the world, frequently relying on one another for every emotional need, while exchanging stories, memories, and desires. Lais explains:

> The thing is that in these jobs we become part of the family, more than that, we are the family who is always there. If the elder all of a sudden develops, I don't know, high blood pressure, one starts to panic. When the elder gets sad, I get sad too, even if I try to distract him or her. It's inevitable. We live together. Their pain becomes also my pain a little.

The creation of these strong emotional bonds often entwines itself with another central aspect of these relationships of labor: the construction of the worker as "one of the family" (among others: Huang & Yeoh, 2007; Parreñas 2014; Rollins, 1985; Romero, 1992). This is a construction that is supported not only by the employers who need to transform perfect strangers into fictive family members able to replace them in the provision of eldercare but also, as Lais points out, by the workers.

This feeling of closeness is also reflected in the language that most of the workers adopt when talking to or about the person in their care. Most of them refer to the elders either as *Nonno* or *Nonna* (grandpa or grandma), exactly in the same way as a family member would do. By using these terms the workers not only take on the role employers designed for them, but they also make sense of their own work. Deborah, a Peruvian worker in her 40s, explains:

> I love this job because with Grandma I feel as if I was with my own grandma. She needs company, affection. . . They need us because the family can't always be there, they have their own work.

Not all the workers, however, enjoy this kind of emotional tie. Maria Julia says:

> Looking after the elders is an exhausting job. It's not like working in an office where at 6 you close the door and you go home. This is a never-ending job. One can do this only for money because it is a very difficult job.

Afina talks about the elders in her care with a lot of affection, but also describes how the relationship is fraught with an inequality in power:

> I'm very happy to work here; they don't consider me simply as a *badante* [elder caretaker]. They consider me as a niece, as one of the family. I always eat with them, they ask me what I want to eat, and we really

> have a strong relationship. I grew up learning to respect my elders, and it works, I respect them and they respect me. I simply had to get used to their needs and behave as they want me to.

While Afina reiterates, like most of the women do, the strong relationship that this work generates, she also highlights the fact that to get along and feel part of the family she has to learn how to please them. It therefore becomes evident that the relationship, although affectionate and even respectful, is certainly not on equal terms. She is made to feel as if she is one of the family, but she is still a *paid* family member, and therefore she needs to learn the rules and to follow them.

ONE OF US...

As the elders and their families begin to consider the worker a member of the family a few tendencies seem to emerge. On the one hand, as many scholars have pointed out (among others Anderson, 2000; Enloe, 1989/2000; Romero, 1992), the family, who is the real employer in these work relations, will attempt to extract more work from the worker with no subsequent pay raise, mirroring the notion that female family members have always performed this job gratuitously. The worker's daily tasks as well as her responsibilities will tend to increase with time. On the other hand, making the worker feel as if she is one of the family allows employers to obtain a stronger labor control on the worker even when they are not present because the worker is expected to behave as one of them at all times.

Being considered as *one of the family*, however, does not always have a negative effect. In some cases it helps the worker to share her concerns about her own family and the people she has left behind. Afina explains:

> Antonio and Nora now really love me, they trust me, they treat me as if I was their own daughter . . . and they are very sentimental. They want to know everything about me: what happened, why I had to leave my country. When they see that I'm sad or worried they always ask me. . . . Antonio even gave me his own phone card to call home, to call my mother and daughter. He said, "You don't have money right now, take it, you need it." They are really good people. This is more than a job. It is collaboration; it is a friendship.

Emotions, as we can see from this quote, work both ways and once the elders become attached to the care provider, their problems become the family problems. It is through the emotional attachment and the sharing of time and stories that home eldercare assistants regain their full dimension as people: people with a past, a present, and a future, people with needs and desires, and people with families to take care of. In this dimension the emotional bond that develops between the elders and their home eldercare assistants becomes the space in which workers become real and the family begins to sympathize with their struggles and difficulties and, in some cases, the workers obtain some level of support and help. However, the relationship between the elders and the home eldercare assistants avoids, in some ways, the maternalism (Romero, 1992) that affects the relationship between employers and domestic workers. Although there is certainly an inequality of power between the elders and the im/migrant workers, the distance that separates them is smaller than the distance that separates the employers and the workers. Both the elders and the workers are marginalized in society and both are extremely vulnerable and dependent on other people.

Most importantly, however, becoming a member of the family allows the worker to obtain greater bargaining power. When the relationship with the elder becomes so strong that the worker becomes irreplaceable, there is a shift in the relationship of power between the employer and the employee. Once the worker becomes the only person who the elders want around, she is no longer the dispossessed immigrant in need, but becomes a valuable and unique asset. It is at this point, and only at this point, that she is able to obtain more control of her own working conditions, her time off, her vacation, and her ability to obtain or maintain a residence permit. This is true for both regular and irregular im/migrants, but it is a particularly important achievement for the irregular worker who, in this way, will secure the support of the family in helping her to obtain legal status—another key element in her ability to achieve better control over her life and her working conditions. In some cases it even allows her to acquire her own domestic worker. Irina recounts:

> A few years ago, after I had already been with Grandma for three years, and a year after my daughters arrived, I decided to leave the job. I wanted to see if I could get my diploma as a nurse recognized in Italy, maybe study some more. I wanted to get an apartment for ourselves, I wanted to live with my daughters, so I spoke with Sara's daughter Anna and I left. Anna hired two other women to fill my place, she was unhappy but she knew that she couldn't do anything about it. Oh my! Grandma didn't last a week. . . . Apparently the day after I left she began to scream all day long, day and night. Her dementia was out of control. She didn't want to see anybody. She was angry at everybody and particularly at Anna because she thought that it was her fault that I'd left. I tried to come visit once but she didn't let me in. She kept screaming, "Go away, you betrayed me, you left me." After a week of that behavior Anna called me and said, "Listen I know that for you the family is everything, but. . . I really need you to come back, otherwise I don't think that my mother will make it through this. . ." So I spoke to the girls and told them that I couldn't do this to the family who had welcomed me in this country, who had helped me to

> obtain the residency permit, and who had also helped them to rejoin me. So, we all went back to live with Sara. Since then the job has improved quite a bit. . . Anna has hired another girl so that I can have more time off to spend with my family, and because she does most of the cleaning, I can spend more time with Grandma. I take care of her physical and mental well-being.

At the same time because Irina is considered a member of the family, she finds herself fulfilling all sorts of tasks for Irina and Anna's family including walking Anna's daughter's dog, watering her plants, cleaning the building stairs, and returning earlier from her free weekend to make sure that the other woman was taking good care of Grandma. Irina says:

> Yes, even if there is another person, I feel that I'm responsible for Sara all the time, even when I'm away. This Sunday for example I was off work but Grandma had a stroke. Anna was away for the weekend and the other woman didn't know what to do, so I left my daughters with their father, gave up my day off and came back to take care of Sara. The woman did other things while I stayed with Grandma, because this is what I have to do. When grandma is involved I don't look at the clock; I stay night and day, and it's my duty.

In some cases the process of becoming part of the family is reciprocated and the elder becomes part of a new international family. Marikit, for example, recounts:

> Grandma is really sensitive, she has a great heart. All my relatives can come and visit me here at work. All of them, no exception. . . . When it's Grandma's birthday I organize a party for her and invite all my relatives, we have a great relationship. She is the grandma of everybody in my family. When I tell her "Grandma, today my cousin is coming for lunch," she asks me, "Oh, good, what should we prepare for her?" She is really nice and loving. I saw my other cousins and their elders are not as nice. In my family five of us work as elder care workers but only two of us, my aunt and I, are able to take their families to their jobs. The others can't. When somebody comes to visit from the Philippines, I always bring them here to see my grandma and every time I tell her that we are going to have a guest she makes sure that we have something good to offer them. Grandma has become part of our culture (laughs).

The strong relationship between cared for and caregiver that makes these jobs bearable, if not pleasant for some, is suffocating for others, at least in the live-in dimension of the job. Petronela, 33 years old, a Romanian woman, remembers:

> The problem is that once the elder gets used to you he or she doesn't want anybody else. The family doesn't want anybody else in their house and that makes it hard because you can't alternate, you can't leave them with anybody else and it is exhausting if you work 24 hours a day. Last year I asked for two weeks vacation and they gave me only one because they wouldn't know what to do with Grandpa for two weeks and they didn't want me to bring in a replacement. They didn't want anybody new in the house.

The families of the elders contribute to this emotional entanglement because once they develop a trusting relationship with the worker they become reluctant to let her go, even for a short time. It is important to remember that for a large number of elders and their families the idea of accepting a stranger, and even more, a foreigner, is not a decision taken lightly. For the elders, coming from a generation not used to the presence of im/migrant and often from a class position that never involved having domestic help in the house, sharing the space with a perfect stranger coming from a different culture is a difficult adjustment. For the families of the elders, the adjustment may not be as great as that required of the elder, but it still requires them to defer responsibilities and open a private space, both physical and emotional, to somebody who is often chosen simply because they are female and relatively inexpensive. Once these decisions are made and the workers prove trustworthy, it becomes difficult for the families to let them go or to introduce yet another person into their homes.

In some cases the worker has to do even more than become a family member; sometimes she has to become the family itself. In this sense home eldercare assistance is not only different from domestic work but it is also different from baby-sitting and nanny jobs. Although babysitting requires the same amount of love, patience, and care as home eldercare assistance, with nannies and babysitters there is always the supervision and the presence, even if only in terms of rules to follow, of the parent. The worker is only the second in command; she is not the one who makes important decisions but most likely she follows the instructions of the parent. In the case of home eldercare assistance, instead, there are many instances in which the full responsibility of the elder falls upon the worker. Maria Elena, a Chilean woman in her mid 40s, explains:

> The gentleman I work for in the morning never had kids. It is the family of his brother that cares for him: his sister-in-law or his niece, but sometimes I feel that they do it only because there is money in it. They don't really care about him; there is no affection.... I am the one who takes care of him, who gives him his medication, who calls the doctor if there is an emergency. Sometimes I feel bad, I feel alone, overwhelmed... too much responsibility.

Different reasons lead to this outcome: it may be because some families live away from their elders, or because they believe that their lives are already difficult enough to manage without the burden of an ailing relative. In some cases, however, even when families are actively involved in the well-being of their elders, they become too scared to watch their parents decay and are unable to face it first hand. Luz recounts:

> The offspring often do not want to accept that their mother and father have changed. They show fear; it is difficult for them to deal with their parents' demise. I worked for an elderly lady for eight years, until she died. During these eight years I saw her suffering, her decay, her shit. She had seven children but I was the only one that wanted to be with her.

The difficulties inherent in the slow demise of these elders are also reflected in the words of one employer, Belinda, whose mother, 80 years old, is afflicted by diabetes, Parkinson's disease, and Alzheimer's disease:

> My mother lives in her own home with a *badante* (elder caretaker), but my sister and I alternate the weekends and, honestly, during those weekends that I spend with her I feel like I'm dying a little too.

Other families that are in charge of more distant relatives such as aunts or uncles do not feel committed enough to provide their presence and care; Luz continues:

> I work now for a very rich family and they tell me "Luz, tell us what you need to take care of our aunt and we'll give it to you. We simply want her to be well dressed and well cared for, we can't lose face in front of our friends." In this case they are not scared; it's not that they don't want to see. They simply don't want to commit to her. We would never behave like this in the Philippines.

The absence of the family has a double effect on the workers. On the one hand they may feel overwhelmed by the responsibilities, but at the same time it may also be the source of great pride, satisfaction, and power. Viviana recalls:

> I was the only one there. Let me just give you an example. One summer, the lady I was working for had decided to let herself die. She was sad because her son was distant and would never come to see her, so she stopped eating. She didn't eat for a full month. After that I took her to the hospital, to see a geriatric doctor. They did some blood tests but nothing happened. Things started to get worse to the point that if I gave her a spoon of water she would throw up. So I took her to the emergency

> room and I thought, I can't assume all this responsibility, and I decided to call her son. I explained all that was going on and do you know what he told me? He said, "You're doing well. Just ask the doctor for some syrup to make her eat. You take care of this," and, honestly, I felt terrible. I felt terrible because in those months I had grown close to that lady and I couldn't believe that a son would behave that way. I hung up and since that moment I took it upon myself to nurse her back to life. . . . This happened in July. In October she was back sitting at the table eating like a proper girl. It was an incredible satisfaction.

Viviana's engagement in her work is not uncommon and shows how the emotional ties that this job engenders make workers go well beyond their line of duty and certainly well beyond their wages.

These close relationships are not exclusive to the cases in which the families are absent. In some cases the worker can become the primary person to care for the elder, even in the presence of loving family members, due to the knowledge the workers acquire of the elder through their daily routines. Irina clarifies:

> I'm the one who is in charge of Grandma. It is five years that I have lived with her, day and night and when something happens to her, Anna, her daughter asks me what to do. In this house I am the person in charge. If Grandma doesn't feel well, I am the one who takes charge of the situation. And this is what I like about this job, the fact that my professionalism is reflected in how Grandma feels. Certainly I clean the house because everybody needs to live in decent conditions, but my job is Grandma and that job I do with pleasure and love.

In both cases the workers admit that it is *being in charge* that can make these jobs satisfactory and even rewarding. Lais says:

> I think that this job can offer a lot of satisfaction. One because the elders are always happy to see you and two because after a while they tend to trust you more than they trust their own offspring.

In other words while these jobs are certainly difficult in terms of hours, wages, working conditions, and emotional strain, they can also offer a certain amount of satisfaction because the workers are never alienated from the object of their labor. What the workers do—the care and the attention they put into their work—is reflected in the physical and emotional condition of the elders in their care. The better the elders feel both physically and emotionally, the greater the satisfaction for the worker. Unfortunately, however, in most cases due to age and physical condition the elder's health tends to worsen and when that happens the worker perceives it as a personal failure. In the previous chapter

I mentioned Luz's experience and how difficult it was for her to accept Nora's suicide attempt, to the point that she became ill. But even when the situation is not as extreme, workers have great difficulties in dealing with the progressive loss of functions of the elders, and eventually with the elder's death. Lais explains:

> There is nothing bad about this job, really, I do like it. The only difficult moments I can recall was when the lady I was working for couldn't recognize me anymore. It wasn't her fault, it was the disease. She wasn't able to recognize her own family. Nevertheless, I couldn't help it. I was really upset, it hurt me that she couldn't recognize me. I cried a lot in those days, particularly because I felt helpless.

Death is at center stage in these work relations. Most of the workers have experienced a loss at least once or twice in their careers and each time the experience has scarred them. Afrodita recalls:

> It is hard, even now after months because I still live in the same building, and when I walk past her door and my son asks me about Grandma . . . for a while I had her voice in my ears every day, I could hear her calling my name "Diiiita, Diiiita." When she went to the hospital because she was in pain, she was screaming the entire time and she died with my name on her lips. When her daughter and I arrived at the hospital the doctor asked us who was "Drita" and her daughter answered "Drita is the woman who took care of her" and the doctor looked at me and said "Look, she died calling your name, she called you with her last breath." And I cried and I cried because . . . she was like a real Grandma to me. I loved her and she loved me.

The length of the working relations coupled with the intimacy that develops in these jobs makes dealing with the loss difficult and although most workers swear each time to having learned a lesson, death always catches them off guard. For this reason some workers, like Aline, choose to abandon this line of work:

> I had to stop working as a home eldercare assistant because it was too painful. It was too difficult to keep getting close to people who sooner or later would die. I had to learn how to put up a barrier and the only way to do it was to change jobs, so I switched to domestic work. Cleaning houses is exhausting but at least there are no emotional involvements.

The death of the elders is also a difficult time for the worker because it ends her life as it was and it terminates her role in the family. Death is a time at which all the contradictions inherent in these jobs come to the forefront and the emotional and economic aspects that were muddled and intertwined up to this point suddenly become manifest and disentangled. It is common for families in times of mourning to retrench and close ranks, and, in some cases, this means excluding the worker from the grieving process. The acquired family member is suddenly returned to the role of an unattached im/migrant worker. Madeline recounts:

> When the elders die it is a terrible time. When the grandma I was working for died, I went to see the family and the only thing they were able to tell me was "What are you doing here today? We are not going to pay you. You know that right?" The daughter sent me away without understanding that I was mourning as much as she was. The day of the funeral, when they were going to drive her body to the mountains where she was from, I said, "I'm coming too" and the daughter didn't want to take me. It was her husband who told her that I had the right to go. Then the daughter said, "and how is she going to get there?" and I said "with your car" and I sat in it. The husband laughed and that's how I got to go to the funeral.

But even when the families understand and support the workers' grieving, the workers still have to face the loss of their job, sometimes their lodging, and the comfort of their daily routines, and again face precariousness and uncertainty. Afina summarizes these feelings:

> I hope that Antonio and Eleonora [the elders she assists] will live a long time because my daughter has to finish her studies, she learns so well. . . . She is seventeen now and I hope she will be able to continue on to the university.

Losing the job also means having to start the process all over again: finding a new job, entering the private realm of another family, getting used to their different needs and desires, and once again getting emotionally attached to a person who eventually, sooner rather than later, will die. Elvire explains:

> Starting a new job is always very difficult, but then after a while you get used to it, you even get to like and love the people you work for. The problem is that when they die you have to start all over again and, not only, you also never know when you'll find a new job. It can even take up to a year to find a new place. In my life I can never make long-term programs because I never know what will happen tomorrow.

Elvire's words emphasize the fact that each of these jobs is designed to please one specific person at one specific time and that the skills acquired for one job are not necessarily transferable to the next. A new job means learning everything all over again: how the elders like their house cleaned, what they like to eat and how they want it cooked, what makes them happy, how to quiet them down, and what medications are needed and when. Each elder has a different set of ailments, different psychological requirements, and different expectations. Elvire also illustrates the extreme precariousness inherent in these jobs and how difficult it is for workers to be able to make long-term plans for their lives, not only in terms of wages, but also for their immigrant status.

Although there are some jobs that can last for years, the majority of them last between 1 and 24 months, hardly enough time to give workers a sense of stability, as Gisela, a Peruvian worker in her early 50s, states:

> I worked twice with the elders, with a lady for a year and with a gentleman for seven months. Unfortunately they both died. And each time I had to start all over again. Something always happened, either they got sicker and died, or the family put them in a structure and I wasn't needed any longer. For example a week ago I started a new job with a lady who was 92 years old. She needed help because she had had a stroke, but she died after two days and I had to start looking all over again.

Precariousness and the lack of a long-term future are also reasons why ethnic groups that have a stronger and longer presence in Italy, such as the Filipinas, tend to avoid these jobs. As Luz explains:

> People of my ethnic group work as home eldercare assistants only to get a foothold in this country because this job has no future. We tend to prefer jobs like custodians or domestic workers because the elders inevitably die.

For some workers, however, death may have a completely different meaning than loss and precariousness. For some, death becomes a deadline that is dreaded and longed for at the same time. Irina, Marikit, Luz, and Rahxma, for example, have each been working at the same job and with the same person for a period of time that ranges from 5 to 8 years. During these years they have developed such a bond with the elder in their care that they have tied their lives and their future to them. Each of them has, in fact, decided to remain on the job while their "grandma" is alive. This decision, although not guaranteeing any certainty for the future, in effect puts their lives on hold—a hold whose length is not quantifiable. And although their position may at first glance appear not to involve precariousness, because it guarantees them a certain stability and the opportunity to save money, it is actually precariousness at its extreme. It is not because the women are afraid of losing their jobs; on the contrary, although they may actually hope for a reprieve at times, the uncertainty, the unknown does not allow them to make any plans for the future or make any long-term decisions. Marikit talks about these conflicting feelings:

> I have been with Grandma for seven years, and I'm not saying that I wish for her to die, but I'm going to stay with her until she dies and then, that will be the time to change job. I am not looking forward to it because that would mean that Grandma has to die, but at the same time . . .

In these cases the emotional relationship developed with the elder tends to become an emotional trap, a tender web that imprisons workers for an unpredictable amount of time. In this case, death is viewed in an ambivalent way: on the one hand it brings loss, grieving, and displacement, but at the same time, when it finally comes, it may also offer the opportunity for a new life.

Aside from the emotional ties and the satisfaction drawn from having control over how the job is done, there are other reasons why immigrant women find a certain level of satisfaction in working with the elders. Some enjoy this job more than others for cultural reasons. Madeline explains:

> I prefer to work with the elders rather than with children purely for a cultural reason. In my culture children are certainly important, but they don't matter as much because they haven't done anything yet. Instead, the elders are more important because they have done things in their lives and for that they have more value.

This is a notion that is supported by Luz:

> For me this job is like a vocation. For us in the Philippines the elders are precious. I learned with my grandmother. I was raised with these values and I still enact them. I like to help people.

Like Madeline, Luz draws from her cultural background the guiding principles of her relationship with the elders, but to them she also adds a personal goal: the desire to help other people. Such a desire is common among the women I interviewed. A large number of them mentioned the importance of feeling needed, of knowing that their work, aside from providing them with much needed wages, does make a difference on a daily basis. Irina explains:

> When I came to Italy I knew that I would have done this job and not another one. I was a nurse in my country, the head nurse of the hospital. I knew that I would have never worked in a bar or in a restaurant. This job is much more important.

And Veronica adds:

> I like to help people who are in need. Aside from the material aspect of this job, I do really like to be able to offer affection to these elders. I believe that what we do is important because what we do with these elders who are at the end of their lives is giving them a little tranquility, a little happiness.

Finally, some workers prefer this job over other jobs available to them simply because it offers a nicer pace, a more tranquil way of life. Ligaya, a Filipina woman in her late 30s, explains:

> I prefer to work with the elders because overall for me it is less work. When you work for a family you should always be doing something. Instead with the elders sometimes you go for a walk, sometime you just sit down and chat. They just want your company and I prefer that, particularly because I have a hip problem and I can't move too much.

The majority of the women I interviewed agreed that the job in itself it is not a bad job; what makes it difficult and sometimes unbearable are the working conditions, the lack of freedom, and the unequal power relations between employers and employees.

Overall, the relationships between the elders and the assistants, while certainly challenging due to the exhausting working conditions and the difficulties of dealing with individuals suffering from a progressive loss of function, as well as their emotional neediness, are more balanced in terms of power than the ones between the home eldercare assistants and their real employers, the elders' families. In the first case, the powerlessness and the needs of immigrant women workers lacking families, affection, work, status, and often rights are somewhat counterbalanced by the powerlessness and the neediness of the elders. Certainly power inequalities are not erased in these relationships, but there is more of a sense of mutual responsibility and support. It is for these reasons that the emotional bond often tends to become more important than more material concerns, even to the point of becoming a trap.

THE REAL EMPLOYERS

The same cannot be said about the relationships between home eldercare assistants and their employers, the elders' families. These relationships are fraught with contradictions, are more fragile, and are extremely unequal in terms of power. The families, and not the elders, control the work relations, even if, in many cases, the wages of the workers are actually paid with the pension or the savings of the elders. Daughters, sons, nieces, or nephews are the ones who establish the wages and the working conditions, and because of the tenuous legal positions of the workers, it is largely up to them as to whether the workers' experiences will be positive or negative, or if they will be respected or obliged to work in slave-like conditions. Among the women I interviewed, only one out of 35 had actually signed a formal contract. Even in cases in which the employers were willing to follow all the legal requirements in terms of wages, hours, holidays, benefits, and social security contributions, the actual work agreements remained informal. Eva, a Peruvian worker in her 30s, recounts:

> The elderly lady's daughter is actually my real employer. She and I agreed on the wages and also on the schedule. I start my day at 8:30 am, then right after lunch I have two hours free either to rest or to do what I like. When I have to go run some errands I tell her and either she comes up or she sends one of her kids. It's all very clear but we don't have a real contract, it is simply an agreement between two people and up to this moment everything has gone relatively well.

Many workers, however, mention how the lack of a formal agreement means that their tasks, their hours, and their wages are subject to constant revision. Madeline says:

> As it is employers cannot only hire and fire us at their whim, but they can also change our duties and our status at any time. A person that calls me to look after her mother, her father or her son certainly needs to ask me if I am qualified for that job, but once that is established she should respect my professionalism and that doesn't always happen.

Families can also choose whether to be helpful regarding the workers' immigration status or take advantage of it. Within a short period of time Aline experienced both extremes of behavior from the families:

> My first job was with an elderly lady who was ninety years old. She was difficult but that was not the main problem. The problem was that her family didn't want to pay me enough. So I kept going to the nuns complaining about that and they were able to find me another job. I left her and I went to work for this new family who loved me. However, the family of the elderly lady was angry at me for leaving the job and, knowing that I was in the country illegally, sent the police to my new job. The police didn't arrest me because the family I was working for was relatively powerful and knew people, and they had sort of adopted me, but the police made me leave the job and I found myself in the middle of the street.

The majority of the workers mentioned at least one or two experiences in which families attempted to take advantage of their position as irregular immigrants. Petronela recalls:

> Every time I would ask the family for a small raise they would threaten to send me back to Romania. If it was up to them I would just work for free. They don't understand that I'm here to work, not to solve their problems. If I had to care for somebody for free I would take care of my father. He too is old and he too needs care.

Obtaining a residency permit, however, while certainly being a huge improvement in the workers' lives, does not guarantee an upgrade in the work relations. Employers know all too well that the workers need the job in order to be able to renew it and they also know that informal agreements can be breached at any time. Gisela remembers:

> Families don't always treat you as they should. I just finished a three month job that I left because I couldn't take it anymore. When they hired me they told me that the lady was very quiet and she just needed some company. It wasn't true. She was afraid of the dark and at night she would go crazy. I slept only an hour or two each night for three months. It was a terrible job, I was the third person to try it and I did it only to renew my permit to stay. When I left, instead of giving me the 820 euros[1] we agreed upon they gave me only 620. No explanation. It was the first time that this happened to me and I didn't protest.

The majority of the workers are well aware of their weak position not only as workers but also as im/migrant. Lack of respect was a common theme during the training class at TierraMadre. All of the women believed that in some way or another their work was not adequately recognized and respected by their employers, but at the same time they were not willing to achieve their goals through unity. Certainly there was a desire to become more qualified, more professional, and to see their labor adequately compensated, but at the same time the majority of the women wanted to maintain their ability to bargain according to individual situations. For this reason, even if at a theoretical level there was a desire to fight to improve working conditions, the strategies tended to be, mostly, individualized. Madeline describes:

> We need to present ourselves as workers with skills and knowledge and not as needy. I always explain to my employers that yes, I need to work, but also that I have rights, maybe not as a worker but as a human being. What we do is hard and important work, but often they

> do not respect us. I'll give you an example: I look after a Grandma who, I don't know how, caught lice. Nobody in the family cared to tell me. Luckily I overheard a conversation among the daughters who were saying "but somebody told Madeline that grandma has lice?" and the answer was "no, no." So I told them "sorry but I'm not going to touch Grandma's head any longer" and they got mad at me. So, I left the house went to the pharmacy and bought a medicated shampoo that I paid for with my own money. Then I went back home and I washed both my and Grandma's head and I told her: "Here Grandma, you and I don't deserve that." Once finished, I walked into the living room and handed the pharmacy receipt to her daughters.

The relationships with the employers are not necessarily always negative. Many workers also talked about the profound relationship that they established not just with the elders but also with their families. Irina explains:

> With Anna I always felt at home, she took me under her wing and I feel protected. I know that she tries to solve any problem that may come my way. They pay me well and they helped in all possible ways to reunite my family. True, we work a lot but they pay me as a nurse and we all live here for free. As soon as she was able to she got me a permit of stay. She was very good. With them I really found a family. When I was here alone we would have dinners together and invite friends. I have plenty of Italian friends. I would make Moldavian food and they would help me. Now my family is here and I can't do that any longer but I still feel part of the family. If I have a problem, any problem, I go straight to them.

For others the presence and the constant support of a family member helped them get through the job. Afrodita remembers:

> Thank God Grandma's daughter was always there for me. She always helped me out. She would come every day, morning and evening, because she lived close by and when she noticed that I was nervous, we would talk and she would say "call me when you can't take it anymore." Since then we have remained close friends. Even now, months after the death of her mother, she comes to visit me and I go visit her. Today for example she is going to take my son and me to the seaside with her. We are going to stay there for three weeks at her house. We remained friends because she is like family to me. I behaved well with them and they did the same with me.

In the cases described by both Afrodita and Irina, the job generated not only wages and an emotional attachment to the elder, but also a veritable support network that allowed the im/migrant worker to pass through the bureaucratic difficulties of immigration, to reunite their distant families, and to more easily navigate life in the new country.

CONCLUSIONS

In this chapter I explored the complexities of eldercare work and of the relationships it generates between all the actors involved. What emerges through workers' lived experiences is a job that in itself is not a bad job per se, but one that becomes bad because of the working conditions that it imposes, including the extremely unequal power relations between workers and employers, the absence of workers' protection, the unnecessary burdens imposed by the current immigration law, and the lack of recognition of the importance and value of this work. As Madeline accurately points out:

> What we need is to figure out how to improve this job that in itself is not a bad job because it involves dealing with human beings; what is bad is everything that surrounds it.

The chapter also emphasizes that the emotional attachment developed in these relationships, although certainly overwhelming, is also what makes the job enjoyable. The emotional relationships that the workers develop with the elders in their care have the function not only to tie them to low wages, longer hours, and more work, but also to morally justify and accept a job that, for the most part, they never wanted to do. This same emotional attachment may also, in some cases, be used to gain bargaining power. Once the workers become irreplaceable for the elders or the elders' families, it becomes easier to request help in obtaining better working conditions, better wages, and a residency permit.

Finally, the relationships developed between the elders and the workers are qualitatively different from the ones developed between the families and the workers. At the beginning, the workers need to work harder to gain the confidence of the elders, because of the novelty of the relationship and the fact that for historical, traditional, and cultural reasons Italian elders are not used to the presence of im/migrant workers and are resistant to sharing their private space with strangers. However, once the relationship is established the elders become greatly attached to and very appreciative of the work done by their homecare assistants. Both subjects share a marginal position in contemporary societies, and the acknowledgment that both sides are in need makes them more willing to adjust to and accept one another. On the other hand, the relationships between the families and the workers are often more complex. Although families may more quickly accept im/migrant workers in their houses to obtain brief relief from the burden of care, relationships hardly seem to go beyond the employer/employee roles. Family caregivers will certainly do everything in their power to retain workers who have proved themselves reliable and trustworthy; however, this goodwill, in most cases, disappears with the death of the elder. Unfortunately, relationships between families and the workers are still too fraught with power inequalities based on hierarchies of race/ethnicity, class, and nationality to develop any real solidarity. These relationships are based on "need": on the one hand the need that im/migrant workers have for a job, a place to live, money to send home, and legal status in the country, and on the other hand the need that families have to find somebody willing to provide, for wages, a substitute for a daughter, a son, or a relative. Once the need of the families disappears, with the death of the elder, so does their allegiance to the worker.

NOTE

1 820 euros corresponds to approximately \$924, whereas €620 corresponds to \$698.

8
CONCLUDING THOUGHTS

In this book I have explored how a progressive aging of the population at the global level and a significant extension of the life span in the countries of the Global North are generating a sense of crisis. This expanding need for services is the source of growing concern for many countries around the globe, which are struggling to find a potential solution for this problem—one that has no precedent and that is only destined to grow. To better understand the problems inherent in this development I explored the current organization of eldercare in Italy, a country that has been in the midst of an eldercare crisis for the past 20 years. In Italy the answer to the eldercare crisis has taken the form of home eldercare assistance, an arrangement whereby short-term and long-term care services are bought in the market by families in the form of private and individualized assistance, sometimes with the help of cash provisions provided by the State. These services, which range from live in jobs requiring 24/7 assistance to live out jobs requiring only a few hours of companionship, are, to this day, provided predominantly by immigrant women, less often men, coming from different areas of the world ranging from Latin America to Eastern Europe, from Asia to Africa, for whom the state has made special provisions in terms of immigration law. This book highlights how this organization, which at first glance and based on many public accounts is presented as a simple market solution involving individual families in need of care and im/migrant workers needing jobs, or as "homemade welfare" (Gori, 2002; Iref, 2007) as some scholars describe it, in reality requires the meshing of global, regional, and national processes to come into place.

As pointed out in Chapter 2, this new arrangement of care does not simply reflect idealized notions of care at the familial level but also a widespread neoliberal approach common to many wealthy, postindustrial countries, according to which the growing demand for care and the cost associated with it are better addressed through market-oriented mechanisms and ideologies. This approach, which has transformed the ways in which care is understood, has been translated into the creation, at the welfare level, of cash for care programs that allow care receivers, now conceived of more as consumers than citizens in need of support, to choose the best care they can buy, in the form they prefer, and with the flexibility they need. Although the introduction of cash for care programs has been interpreted in different ways in different countries (Da Roit, 2007, Shutes, & Chiatti 2012; van Hooren, 2012), in Italy, a country where the role of the welfare state was historically limited and in which families were always at the forefront of care provision (Bettio & Plantenga, 2004), the implementation of this program has fundamentally helped to transform Italian elders and their families into employers. In addition, by enacting this program without a clear set of rules on how to use this support and on who to hire, the state has become complicit in the development of an unregulated labor market that seeks to obtain the most labor for the least amount of money.

A similar process is visible in the creation of the labor market of care described in Chapter 3. Italy, in fact, unlike other countries, such as England or the United States, did not have a fully developed market of formal eldercare services to supply families with the care they needed. Instead, the market, starting from the mid-1990s, took the form of im/migrant labor. It was in those years, in fact, that the growing need for eldercare services coincided with the growing presence of both regular and irregular im/migrants in the country shaping the future of home eldercare assistance. This presence, often presented as the result of simple *push* and *pull* explanations or as "people in need coming for a better life," is, instead, the result of complex global, regional, and national transformations that have dislocated a growing number of people from their original communities. These transformations involve, among other things, increasing global inequality, transformations in the global labor market and in the global division of labor, the political and economic disintegration of the Soviet Union, the progressive introduction of a deregulated form of capitalism in many countries of the Global South, and new immigration laws regulating the circulation of people in the European Union. These transformations, which have affected the lives of entire nations and communities, have also transformed the division of labor among men and women, increasingly incorporating women not only in the global labor market but also in migration flows providing more potential laborers for care and domestic jobs. It is due to the mobilization of im/migrant women across the world that reproductive labor is being redistributed regionally and globally (Parreñas, 2001); as a result of these processes Italian families found themselves able to access a new pool of labor, one that differed radically from the Italian one. Im/migrant workers, in fact, often arrive in the countries of destination already burdened by multiple layers of needs: the need to repay the debt accumulated through the migration process, the need to earn wages as quickly as possible in order to make the distance from families and children left behind meaningful, the need to obtain a visa permit, the need to find a place to stay—needs that can be satisfied only by obtaining a job as quickly as possible, often without regard for the wages or the living/working conditions offered. Im/migrant workers, in reality, are not just workers but are first and foremost im/migrants. This means that their work, pay, working conditions, and overall migratory projects are strictly shaped and defined by the immigration policies of the countries of destination. By dividing according to the labels—regular versus irregular, European Union (EU) national versus non-EU, desired versus undesired—immigration policies shape how im/migrants participate in the labor markets, how they integrate into society, and how they design their overall migratory journeys. In addition, specific migration policies such as quotas or amnesties linked to specific occupations also help to channel im/migrant workers into particular jobs or sectors. In the case of Italy an ambiguous immigration policy that combines restrictive policies on the one hand and periodic regularizations on the other hand, coupled with more fluid immigration policies concerning European citizens, has generated, over time, a situation in which im/migrants experience a great deal of variation in terms of legal status, cross border mobility, and migratory projects. These variations, in turn, produce a segmented labor force willing to accept very different wages, working conditions, and living arrangements, making eldercare affordable for families at all income levels, not simply upper middle class families.

To these large processes it is important to add the daily practices that help to transform im/migrants with different backgrounds in terms of education, class, and provenance into the home eldercare assistants desired by Italian families. These practices include, among others, placing severe obstacles in the recognition of foreign educational degrees or diplomas as well as in the reductive representation of im/migrants in the media, in politics, and in society as either criminal or as " less fortunate people in need." Either way they are regarded as something other, distant, and not equal to the Italian population, resulting in an often unspoken, but widespread discrimination against different races, ethnicities, religions, and nationalities. The Italian organization of eldercare, therefore, can be considered "home made" or a simple arrangement between supply and demand, only if we choose to disregard all the global, regional, and national forces that play a part in creating and managing a segmented im/migrant labor force. It is a force whose presence is crucial in satisfying the eldercare needs of most Italian families as well as in providing the welfare state with a cheap and disposable fix to a growing problem.

ITALIAN FAMILIES: FROM CAREGIVERS TO CARE-MANAGERS WITHOUT CHALLENGING THE GENDERED STATUS QUO

Global, regional, and national inequalities are not the only inequalities inherent to home eldercare assistance. Others become apparent once we start to analyze the organization of care in the private sphere. The data collected for this project, in fact, indicate that home eldercare assistance is the area in which Italian families, im/migrant women, and Italian elders come together in extremely unequal relationships of power. Italian women, unable, and often unwilling, to challenge the cultural and economic status quo according to which reproductive work remains a "woman's affair" find themselves crushed by the growing demand for care placed on them, a demand that in the case of eldercare grows and expands overtime often filling every available minute of the day. These demands coupled with structural ones, such as demographic changes, shifts in family structures, and increased and extended participation in the labor market, often make it impossible for women to fulfill all of their care obligations, often pushing them to subcontract some of this care to other women, often im/migrant women. What the interviews reveal is that Italian women come to this decision not to pursue status, better lifestyles, or more satisfactory careers (Anderson, 2000; Hondagneu-Sotelo, 2001; Yeates, 2009), as do many of their counterparts who hire domestic workers or nannies, but rather out of exhaustion and exasperation. Eldercare, in fact, differs from other forms of care because it grows and expands over time. Unlike child care, in which the demands diminish over time, in the case of aging parents or relatives the demand for care increases as physical and cognitive functions deteriorate. It may start with a few hours of companionship, then extend to full days, and then, over time, to full days and nights. It should be mentioned that this extended need for care can engulf families for years and decades on end. In the absence of other forms of support the hiring of an im/migrant worker appears to many as the only possible way to maintain sanity, a balance, the semblance of a normal life, and the ability to find relief from those crushing demands.

Nevertheless, like their counterparts in the United States (Chang, 2000; Hondagneu-Sotelo, 2001; Parreñas, 2001; Wrigley, 1995), in other European countries (Andall, 2000; Anderson, 2001; Gluckmann & Lyon, 2006), and in Asia (Constable, 1997), Italian women, instead of seeking other arrangements, take advantage of previously mentioned inequalities that intersect with gender, race/ethnicity, and religion to find this help and to maintain a gendered status quo at home. This book shows that among other things, Italian employers hire im/migrant home eldercare assistants mostly to maintain an ideal notion of gender roles and family that in contemporary postindustrial society struggles to exist. They do so by attempting to recreate the structure of the extended family, thus incorporating the presence of im/migrant women not as workers but as temporary and fictional *less fortunate family members.* This construction allows Italian women and, by extension, their families to fulfill cultural and traditional requirements, reflecting widely shared ideas about what care for the elders should be. Cultural understandings of care are, in fact, as important as economic and political ones and Italian families, to this day, tend to see eldercare as an extension of family duties, which is better accomplished in the privacy of the home rather than in formal institutions. Furthermore, the construction of im/migrant workers as temporary and fictional *less fortunate family members* allows families first to conceive of the job more as a favor than a real job, second to devalue the tasks performed on the job because they come to be seen simply as an extension of the unpaid work commonly performed in the family, and finally to consider im/migrant women, independent of their background in terms of class, education, and skills, simply as "poor women looking for work." These are processes that, taken together, help contain the cost of labor, secure flexibility, ensure dependability, and a sense of attachment to the elders and the family while at the same time maintaining the workers in a position of vulnerability. This vulnerability, in many cases, forces the workers to accept forms of daily abuse ranging from the refusal to provide them with adequate food, heating, electricity, or privacy to forcing them to abandon their own national, cultural, and religious habits in favor of the Italian ones, and to withstand verbal, physical abuse, and, in some cases, sexual harassment.

Last but not least, this construction allows family caregivers of all social classes to shift their position from "care providers" to "care managers" (Degiuli, 2010), which allows Italian caregivers to delegate the most demeaning aspects of long-term care while retaining moral and spiritual control over the health and the well-being of their relative, thus allowing them to fulfill the traditional filial and parental role.

It is important to point out, though, that the advantage offered by im/migrant women is not limited to the cultural realm but extends to an economic and organizational one. Their presence, in fact, provides families with a low cost, more flexible alternative to institutional structures. Im/migrant women, particularly when irregularly present in the country or engaged in short-term circular migration, are willing to accept very demanding jobs, and, if necessary, full time live-in jobs, for very low wages. In addition, they are willing to work overtime and on weekends, and are easy to dismiss when their labor is no longer needed.

Notwithstanding all these advantages, the interviews with caregivers reveal that not all of them prefer the private market to state-provided services. Although the wealthiest respondents had a clear preference for the private market model and completely disregarded the ability of the state to provide eldercare support, the majority of the respondents wished for a stronger role for the welfare state and for more guidance in navigating the increasing burden of long-term eldercare. In most cases, the decision to turn to the market came only after all other options had been exhausted. Moreover, although most of the respondents commented on the negative aspects connected to the welfare state, such as its extreme rigidity, lack of coordination, and extreme bureaucracy, many of them clearly stated that they longed for a restructured welfare state able to offer them not only financial assistance, but, perhaps most importantly, much better information, services, and different forms of support. Although the interview sample for this project is too small to provide generalizations for the overall population, these insights suggest that not all caregivers want to be transformed into consumers of care and that many still value the role of public services over private ones.

THE WELFARE STATE: MARKET OR BUST

The book also stresses how the presence of im/migrant women who help Italian women create fictional kin networks to maintain a gendered status quo of care provision is functional not only to Italian families but also to the welfare state. The state, in fact, has a great role in generating and supporting models of care that push families to overextend themselves in order to provide care for both children and the elders and consequently to recreate fictional families. As mentioned in Chapter 2, the Italian welfare state is based on what Esping Andersen calls a familialist regime—one that is characterized by limited public services for both children and the elderly, by a shortage of policies that reconcile care and work (Zanatta, 2005), and by a reliance on individual families and their kin network for the provision of care (Burgio et al., 2010; Saraceno, 2003). In fact, even when public provisions are offered it generally consists mostly of financial transfers to the family and only residually of actual care services (Ranci, 2001; Da Roit, 2007). This is further complicated by the fact that the welfare state in Italy is characterized by the presence of multiple actors that includes the state, the regions, the municipalities, and the local health agencies, which in turn control and distribute different forms of funding often without internal coordination (Spano, 2006, p. 20). In addition, this funding, as seen in Chapter 3, is extremely limited and is therefore restricted to a rather small number of families in need.

Therefore, although legislation implemented in the past decade, such as the law 328/2000 and the National Health Plan drafted by the Ministry for Health for 2006–2008, reiterates the importance of maintaining the elders at home and within the family network (Ministero della Salute, 2006, p. 70; Senato Italiano, 2000), in practice little is done at the national level to support families in this endeavor. The pressures on families to be the main care providers is further compounded by a restructuring of the welfare state that has in the past decades reduced the few services already available. Palese and her collaborators (2004), for example, point out that changes in the Italian National Health Service have led to shorter hospital stays and early discharge, causing elderly people to be sent home from the hospital before they are completely healed.

The analysis therefore shows that Italian families are not the only ones to try to replace themselves with im/migrant workers in the provision of care; the Italian welfare state is doing the same.[1] By taking advantage of the presence of im/migrant women and men and their work—a presence and a work guaranteed and disciplined through migration policies—the Italian welfare state is able to reduce the discontent of Italian families, to uphold neoliberal ideologies, and to avoid a full engagement with the growing demand for long-term care.

The presence of im/migrant women workers, therefore, allows for the perpetuation of a fictional reality both at a private level and at an institutional level. It clearly underscores how global processes of dislocation and migration, instead of endangering or undermining nation-states of the Global North[2], actually advantage them.

ELDERCARE: THE MULTIPLE DIMENSIONS OF AGING AND ITS NEEDS

In addition to highlighting the processes that generate these relationships of labor and the inequalities inherent in them this book also provides important insights on the job itself, on its requirements, and on how eldercare differs from other forms of care. A close analysis of the occupation, for example, reveals that home eldercare assistance is a labor-intensive occupation both in terms of productive outputs and emotional labor. The analysis of a typical 24-hour day reveals that during their workday and night home eldercare assistants accomplish a great number of tasks including cooking, cleaning the home, administering medications, cleaning wounds, bathing and dressing the elders, changing diapers, and more. These tasks are often performed in connection with a great deal of emotional labor that ranges from the simple yet demanding need to always display appropriate body and facial expressions to devising complex, strategic tactics to keep the elders satisfied, mentally active, and feeling connected to a larger society. During, often, extremely long workdays, these workers, often constructed as unskilled, take on multiple roles ranging from maid to companion, nurse to spiritual counselor, and entertainer to personal assistant, each one of them requiring a different set of skills and each of them addressing an equally important aspect of care. The goal of each of these tasks is to help the elders to remain comfortable, when possible, to remain mentally and physically active, and to remain connected to families and the larger society for as long as possible. All this is done while also accompanying the elders through the inevitable journey toward death, a journey made of daily losses both at the physical and mental level that often leave the elders in a state of rage and despair. This is difficult work even when the elders are not affected by more serious pathologies such as Alzheimer's and Parkinson's diseases, which according to the women interviewed for this project require two dimensions: a *time of care* and a *time of production*. The first, according to them, is a time that has lost value in wealthy societies. It is a time that does not require constant measurable outputs, but one geared to create a sense of well-being for the person being cared for. It is a time that may involve less cleaning and more listening, less cooking and more singing, and less ironing and more laughing. Time of production, instead, is concerned with productivity—with the constant output of tangible services such as cooking, cleaning, dusting, and ironing. Eldercare work, according to the women who do it, requires both, but for the job to be effective, the former has to be privileged over the latter. In other words, the workers argue, if not for an actual delinking of eldercare from domestic work, for a more defined boundary between the two, one that acknowledges that care should be at the center of these relationships of labor and not at the margins. This is a request that employers, for the most part, struggle to accept not only because they are often concerned with containing the costs of long-term care but also because for most of them it is difficult to quantify, regulate, and, to this day, pay for the intangible, yet fundamental time of care.

Although the words of im/migrant home eldercare assistants are central in providing deeper insights on what long-term care for the elders should be like, they also emphasize some of the dangers inherent to these privatized and individualized relationships of care. Im/migrant women, as illustrated throughout this book, are not hired because of their skills or their experience with elderly people, but rather simply on the basis of their gender, nationality, sometimes religion, and on their willingness to accept low wages and/or demanding conditions of labor. This means that many of the workers hired to provide home eldercare assistants are not necessarily prepared to engage with the complexities of aging, which in turn, means that notwithstanding their good intentions and their best effort, most of the time they may not know that the reason behind the elders screaming, yelling, and accusing them of imaginary crimes is not always just mean spiritedness or racism but, in some cases, full blown dementia or Alzheimer's. They may not know that elderly men and women while looking vulnerable and defenseless are not children, but people with pasts, careers, professions, achievements, and failures and often strong sets of beliefs and preferences not always in tune with the contemporary world, and they may not necessarily know how to treat aging bodies with the dignity and respect that they require. This lack of knowledge and training is dangerous for the workers because it often puts them in extremely difficult situations with nobody to turn to for advice, but also for the elders who may end up being mistreated, endangered, and, in extreme cases, abused by workers. To think that im/migrant women are capable of providing eldercare just because of the skills bestowed on them by their gender or by their culture/nationality is a false proposition that needs to be addressed.

Furthermore, this book highlights how home eldercare assistance, like other forms of care labor, is an incompletely commodified form of labor (Radin, 1996, Himmelweit, 1999), meaning that it is an occupation that involves both market and non market elements. This means that while wages and working conditions play a great part in the definition of *home eldercare assistance,* emotional ties do too. The lived experiences of the workers reveal that *home eldercare assistance* is a job that in itself is not necessarily a bad job, but one that becomes bad because of the working conditions that it imposes, such as the extremely unequal power relations between workers and employers, the absence of workers' protection, the unnecessary burden imposed by the current immigration law, and the lack of will to recognize the importance and value of this work. Certainly it is true that workers may offer a positive description of the job in order to make sense of their downward social mobility (Parreñas, 2001) or to resist the stigma attached to this profession (Stacey, 2005), but some workers honestly seem to appreciate some aspects of the job, particularly the ones that provide them with the notion of being *needed* and *appreciated,* of knowing that what they were doing has a greater meaning than simply providing wages. And, as demonstrated in this book, eldercare is necessary work; without it human beings would not be able to deal with the daily limitations generated by progressive loss of cognitive and physical function and to age and die with dignity. Home eldercare assistance is something that belongs to all of us because in the journey toward decline and, eventually, death that the elder experiences we see our own journey. However, home eldercare assistance in its current form is not only concerned simply with the reproduction of life or in this case with the end of life, it is also concerned with the reproduction of an ideal family that no longer exists, with a notion of femininity that no longer exists. This is where the job becomes no longer sustainable because to provide these elements employers need to find women who are willing to become captives of the home, not their own homes, but of somebody else's home, and the only way to do that is to exploit their vulnerabilities.

Therefore, in order to provide a dignified experience for both home eldercare assistants and the elders in their care it is crucial to distinguish between work and exploitation, between ideals of care and the practice of care. It is important to understand that care can be effectively provided by a paid member of the workforce who is not a family member and to respect and trust that the care provided will be as good and, in some cases, even better than that provided by unpaid family members. This is possible for many reasons: first there is no history between the paid careworker and the elder. The relationship is not laden with years of family history, conflicts, and personal turmoil that often tend to complicate and endanger the relationship of care. Second, the careworker is not as personally invested in the aging and decline of the elder as a family member may be. The progressive decline of the elders is not as hurtful for the worker as it could be for a wife, a husband, a son, or a daughter, and this distance, although difficult to accept at the beginning, in the long run provides the elders with more freedom. Third, as already mentioned, the emotional bond that emerges between the worker and the elder, even if complex and contradictory, is real and has consequences for both parties involved. In fact, it is not uncommon to hear of workers who have been included in the elders' wills or of workers who have chosen to stay on the job until the death of the elders, therefore tying their lives to the lives of their wards. The real challenge therefore, both in Italy and in all countries that are experiencing a growing need for long-term care, will be to understand, develop, and value the bonds that emerge in these relationships rather than to use them to extract more labor from already vulnerable workers.

A DIFFERENT WAY TO THINK ABOUT AGING

In addition to providing us with a deeper understanding of the current organization of care in Italy, the analysis of home eldercare assistance provides us with important insights on what a new more equitable way to think about aging and the growing need for long-term care should look like well beyond Italy. Chapter 1 of this book shows that aging is not a *natural* process, rather one that is greatly influenced by technological, economic, political, and cultural developments that in different combinations and with different timing in diverse geographic areas first helps to reduce the mortality and then the fertility of the population. In addition, it is a process that is further enhanced by medical technologies that, in recent years, have been able to greatly extend, particularly in wealthy countries of the Global North, the life span of many men and women. The result is an older population that lives a longer life. While these achievements have been celebrated, they have also created some side effects. The people who live longer, in fact, are not always able to do so in perfect health. Instead they often require increased medical support, nursing assistance, emotional and physical care, and progressively higher amounts of supervision. These side effects, however, are not addressed by the same mechanisms that have created them; instead, for the most part, they are passed on to individuals and/or their families as if they were their own responsibility. Through this process a societal, collective development is transformed into an individual one sending individuals and families scrambling for affordable, flexible, and manageable forms of care support, which often ends up being provided by vulnerable and unskilled im/migrant workers. The result of this process is the creation of inequities: for the families who are pressed to provide a solution to this problem and to contribute to them in economic, emotional, and temporal forms; for the elders who are transformed from dignified human beings into simply a burden and whose care may not always be adequate; and for the workers who are often underpaid, exploited, and unappreciated. I argue, instead, that in order to effectively address these problems we need to reverse the trend and to bring these issues back into the collective and societal terrain.

We currently live in a world in which all our attention is dedicated to the production of profit, the increase of gross domestic products (GDPs), and the measurement of outputs, but little attention is dedicated to the reproduction of society at all its levels. While macrostructures increasingly acknowledge and take ownership of the productive world, the reproductive world is pushed more and more to the individual level and is increasingly hidden from sight as if it was something slightly dirty. The reproduction of human beings is certainly a little dirty, messy, complicated, and often unrewarding, both economically and in terms of societal recognition, nevertheless, it remains crucial to the existence of society and to the actual reproduction and maintenance of the productive system at the core of neoliberal thinking. Children will be future workers, whereas elderly people were the workers of yesterday. All of us are sick and disabled at different times in our lives. Care and reproduction are important sites where most people's lives actually happen, unpaid work is produced, profit is extracted, and emotions and affection are generated. Hiding the reproductive world from sight and from our collective responsibility is a choice, not an inevitable state of affairs. It is possible to behave otherwise. It is possible and, in my opinion, it should be a duty to bring the reproductive world back into sight and use our collective knowledge and expertise to support it and make it thrive. Care needs to be brought back to the center of our societies instead of being pushed to the margin and it needs to be addressed not simply as a burden or an added cost, but as an integral aspect of our society; it should be supported by well-thought-out resources and the creation of reliable services, which, in turn, would generate the creation of much needed jobs and the creation of a professional workforce valued and respected by society at large. In Italy, for example, some Italian scholars (among others Gori, 2002; Ranci, 2001; Zanatta, 2005) have suggested the creation of a social market of care called a "social market" of services. According to this model the welfare state would provide, either directly or indirectly through supervised outsourcing, a number of more targeted and specific eldercare services created on the basis of families' needs. These services, no longer limited only to the most disadvantaged sectors of the population, would be made available to all strata of the population, who in exchange will contribute to them in different amounts according to income. The provision of services regulated by the welfare states would provide families with the help they need while, at the same time, discouraging them from pursuing informal and individualized care arrangements. Although this system may not be applicable to all countries, due to different beliefs concerning the role of welfare states, it provides a blueprint to think about care as a social endeavor instead of an individual one.

In addition, we need to bring into the discussion gender and its relationship to care. Up to this point the provision of care has been and continues to be predominantly a woman's affair. This is true in Italy, in the United States, and in many other countries around the world. This also needs to change. We need to emerge from the societal discussion with a reconfiguration of care that moves away from the stalled revolution described by Hochschild (1989) in which women have entered the labor market and taken on the same breadwinner responsibilities that men have, although men did not take on the same responsibilities in the home. Just recently the *New York Times* released the results of a study conducted by the American Time Use Survey that shows that even when unemployed, men do not perform the same amount of housework that women do (*New York Times*, January 6, 2015). This current system only produces, as many scholars have pointed out, more inequality among women from different races, ethnicities, nationalities, and social classes.

We need to emerge from our societal discussion with a clear understanding of the fact that economic reality no longer matches current gendered expectations. This is true both in the countries of the Global North and of the Global South. As shown, both in Chapters 1 and 2, women are increasingly becoming co-breadwinners, and, in many cases, the main breadwinners not only for themselves and for their families but often for entire communities and nations. Their work is now central not only for familial reproduction but also for supporting national economies, stalling GDPs, and alleviating expanding poverty, due, among other things, to botched reforms implemented by the International Monetary Fund (IMF) and the World Bank. It is time to acknowledge that economic, political, and social realities no longer match gender roles and gendered expectations. The discussion about gender, therefore, should no longer rest on the question "Can women have it all?" but rather should be centered on answering "How can we make sure that women are no longer asked to do it all?" It is crucial that at this historical conjuncture when the demands for care continue to grow we engage in a societal discussion aimed at acknowledging these new realities and exploring and supporting changes in static and inflexible formulations of femininity and masculinity. Men can become good care providers in the same way in which women can become excellent Prime Ministers. Which leads us to my third point: care needs to be transformed from a devalued practice provided for free into a valuable, fairly rewarded, and highly appreciated activity that is valued as much as creativity and invention. The ability to care is not an extension of gendered beings, rather it is the result of carefully refined and developed skills. Proper caring, in fact, requires sensibility, attention, imagination, creativity, and empathy because care is not just an object of policy making, but, as Williams and Brennan (2012, p. 356) pointed out, it is a "set of social relations that involve power and dependency and affective, intimate, and ethical practices of love, duty, and obligation."

I am quite aware that a societal discussion may be difficult to undertake and that the results may be contradictory, uneven, and difficult to enforce, but it is something that we, as a society, can no longer avoid. The market may provide solutions for the people who have the means to access them, but it does not provide a cultural framework to think about and address the changes we are experiencing in contemporary societies. It is crucial to bring these issues to the forefront of our lives and to develop new ways of thinking about care, ones that no longer push it to the margins and in the hands of the most vulnerable subjects, but that instead embrace its ability to transform society and our relationships in the process.

NOTES

1 Ambrosini (2015) defines the work provided by irregular im/migrant workers in the care labor market as the "invisible welfare."

2 See current discussion on immigration in Europe.

APPENDIX 1—INTERVIEWS WITH CURRENT OR FORMER HOME ELDERCARE ASSISTANTS

Origin of Contact	Name	Nationality	Age	Current Profession	Taped
Tierra	Afina	Romania	38	Eldercare	Yes
Tierra	Afrodita	Albania	38	Eldercare	Yes
Apidad	Aline	Brazil	35	Geriatric social worker	No
Tierra	Beatriz	Peru	32	Eldercare	No
Tierra	Carmen	Ecuador	26	Unemployed	No
Friends	Claudia	Peru	28	Domestic worker	No
Friends	Dalisay	Philippines	28	Domestic worker	No
Tierra	Deborah	Peru	Early 30s	Unemployed	Yes
Benevolentia	Ecaterina	Romania	51	Unemployed	No
Tierra	Elizaveta	Moldavia	45	Eldercare	Yes
Tierra	Elodia	Peru	Early 50s	Eldercare	No
Tierra	Elvire	Ivory Coast	33	Unemployed	No
Tierra	Eva	Peru	Late 20s	Eldercare	Yes
Benevolentia	Gisela	Peru	35	Unemployed	No

(continued)

Origin of Contact	Name	Nationality	Age	Current Profession	Taped
Benevolentia	Gladys	Peru	55	Librarian/ baby sitter	No
Friends	Irina	Moldova	38	Eldercare	Yes
Benevolentia	Isabela	Romania	Early 50s	Unemployed	No
Church	Lais	Brazil	Mid 40s	Eldercare	Yes
Apidad	Leilah	Morocco	22	Unemployed	Yes
Filipino Community	Ligaya	Philippines	39	Domestic worker	No
Tierra	Lucha	Peru	51	Domestic worker	No
Tierra	Luminita	Romania	Mid 40s	Unemployed	Yes
Filipino Community	Luz	Philippines	40	Eldercare	No
Tierra	Madeline	Congo	40	Eldercare	No
Tierra	Maria Elena	Chile	Early 40s	Eldercare	Yes
Apidad	Maria Julia	Peru	38	Unemployed	Yes
Filipino Community	Marikit	Philippines	Late 20s	Eldercare	Yes
Benevolentia	Marisela	Peru	19	Unemployed	No
Benevolentia	Petronela	Romania	33	Unemployed	No
Tierra	Rahxma	Somalia	32	Eldercare	Yes
Benevolentia	Teresa	Ecuador	38	Cultural mediator	No
Tierra	Venera	Albania	28	Eldercare	Yes
Tierra	Veronica	Peru	47	Domestic worker	Yes
Tierra	Viviana	Peru	Early 40s	Domestic worker	Yes
Benevolentia	Zahra	Morocco	Mid 30s	Cultural mediator	No

APPENDIX 2—INTERVIEWS WITH FAMILY CAREGIVERS WHO CARE FOR DISABLED ELDERS

Name	Relationship to Elder	Eldercare Assistant	Elders' Pathologies	Future Goals
Arianna	Niece	No	Broken leg, mentally lucid	Keeping her in her house by hiring an assistant
Belinda	Daughter	Yes	Prostate cancer, not very lucid	Keeping him at home, increasing the hours of an assistant
Benedetta	Daughter	Yes, live in	Alzheimer's disease, Parkinson's disease, diabetes	Keeping her in her house as long as possible
Bettina	Daughter	No longer	Senile dementia	Institutionalize her
Bruno	Son	Thinking about it	Alzheimer's disease	Keeping him at home by hiring an assistant
Carla	Daughter	No	Physically disabled, mentally lucid	Keeping her at home with no external help
Claudia	Daughter	Yes, two	Senile dementia	Keeping her at home as long as possible
Cosimo	Son	Yes, 8 hours a week	Broken femur, mentally lucid	Keeping him at his house

(continued)

Name	Relationship to Elder	Eldercare Assistant	Elders' Pathologies	Future Goals
Costanza	Daughter	Yes, full time	Broken femur	Institutionalize her
Gaia	Daughter	No	Relatively well	Institutionalize her
Giulia	Wife	Yes, 3 hours a day	Alzheimer's disease	Keeping him at home as long as possible
Marina	Daughter-in-law	No	Circulatory dysfunctions	Keeping him at home as long as possible
Martina	Daughter	No, but they are planning on it	Senile dementia	Keeping him at his house as long as possible
Matilde	Daughter	No, but they would like it	Senile dementia	Keeping him at home with his wife as long as possible
Maurizia	Daughter	Yes, two of them	Senile dementia	Keeping her in her house as long as possible
Nicola	Son	No, they had a bad experience	Alzheimer's disease	Institutionalize him
Orazio	Son	Yes, live-in	Alzheimer's disease	Keeping her in her home as long as possible
Paride	Husband	No, but hoping to hire one	Alzheimer's disease	Keeping her at home as long as possible
Piera Silvana	Daughters	No, but they are considering it	Alzheimer's disease	Keeping her in her house as long as possible
Porzia	Daughter	No	Anal cancer, unable to walk after a broken femur	Keeping her at her house as long as possible
Quinto	Son	Yes, during the day	Alzheimer's disease	Keeping her in her house with her husband as long as possible
Sabina	Daughter	Yes, in the morning	Alzheimer's disease, disability	Keeping them in their house as long as possible
Serafina	Sister	No, but they are hoping to	Broken leg	Keeping her at home as long as possible
Stella	Mother and father	No, they are hoping to	None, aside from old age	Keeping them in their house as long as possible
Vanna	Mother	Yes, two	Parkinson's disease, senile dementia	The mother does not want to go into an institution
Vilma	Mother	No, hoping to	Depression, broken leg	Keeping her at home as long as possible

APPENDIX 3—INTERVIEWS WITH CULTURAL MEDIATORS OF TIERRA, APIDAD, AND BENEVOLENTIA AND FOLLOW-UP INTERVIEWS OF 2011

Interviews with Cultural Mediators

Name	Organization
Pilar Flores	Tierra
Consuelo Aguilar	Tierra
Martina Ferrero	Tierra
Sister Ortensia Sivieri	Benevolentia
Caterina Zamboni	Apidad

Follow up Interviews 2011

Name	Position	Organization
Pilar Flores	Cultural Mediator	Tierra
Fabrizia Ierato	Carework Committee	Tierra
Martina Ferrero	Carework Committee	Tierra
Elisabetta Bora	Carework Committee	Tierra
Sandra Santini	Omitted to protect privacy	Trade Union
Roberto Santoro	Director	Temporary Agency

(continued)

Name	Position	Organization
Alessandra Marellli	Home Eldercare Assistants Training Module Director	City of Turin
Stefano Albertelli	Home Eldercare Assistants Training Module Operator	City of Turin
Paola Giacomelli	Mediator between families and workers	Social Cooperative
Roberta Salini	Mediator between families and workers	Social Cooperative

REFERENCES

Agostini, C., Longobardi, E., & Vitaletti, G. (2012). Donne Migranti. Quali opportunità per il nostro paese? *L'Economia dell'Immigrazione*, 0(2), 2–7. Available at http://www.fondazioneleonemoressa.org/rivista/flm/2/rivistaFLM-2.pdf. Accessed on June 14, 2013.

Alden, S. (2011). *Socially Active Older Adults Have Slower Rates of Health Declines*. Center for Advancing Health. Available at http://www.cfah.org/hbns/2011/socially-active-older-adults-have-slower-rates-of-health-declines. Accessed April 20, 2013.

Albert, I., & Ferring, D. (Eds.) (2013). *Intergenerational Relations: European Perspectives on Family and Society*. Bristol, UK: The Policy Press.

Alemani, C. (2004). Le colf: ansie e desideri delle datrici di lavoro. *Polis*, *1*, 137–164.

Altroconsumo. (2013). Inchiesta sulle case di riposo. Available at http://www.altroconsumo.it/soldi/pensioni/news/case-di-riposo-la-retta-e-un-salasso. Accessed July 1, 2014.

Ambrosini, M. (2001). The Role of Immigrants in the Italian Labour Market. *International Migration*, *39*(3), 61–83.

Ambrosini, M. (2013). *Immigrazione Irregolare e il Welfare Invisibile*. Bologna, Italy: Il Mulino.

Ambrosini, M. (2015). Contracts, emotions, and mutual obligations within Italy's invisible welfare system. In *Employers, agencies, and immigration: Paying for Care*. Farnham, Surrey, UK: Ashgate.

Amott, T., & Matthaei, J. (1996). *A Multi-cultural Economic History of Women in the United States*. Boston, MA: South End Press.

Andall, J. (2000). *Gender, migration and domestic service: The politics of black women in Italy*. Aldershot, UK: Ashgate.

Andall, J. (2004). Le Acli-Colf di fronte all'immigrazione straniera: genere, classe ed etnia. *Polis, 18*(1), 77–106.

Andall, J., & Sarti, R. (2004). Le trasformazioni del servizio domestico in Italia: Un'introduzione. *Polis, 1*, 5–16.

Anderson, B. (1997). Servants and slaves: Europe's domestic workers. *Race and Class, 39*(1), 37–49.

Anderson, B. (2000). *Doing the dirty work? The global politics of domestic labor*. London, UK: Zed Books.

Anderson, B. (2001). Why madam has so many bathrobes: Demand for migrant domestic workers in the EU. *Journal of Social and Economic Geography, 92*(1), 18–26.

Anttonen, A., & Meagher, G. (2013). Mapping marketisation: Concepts and goals. In G. Meagher & M. Szebehely (Eds.), *Marketisation in Nordic eldercare: A research report on legislation, oversight, extent and consequences* (pp. 13–22). Stockholm, Sweden: Stockholm University Press.

Anthias, F., & Lazaridis, G. (2000). Introduction: Women on the Move in Southern Europe. In F. Anthias & G. Lazaridis (Eds.), *Gender and Migration in Southern Europe: Women on the Move* (pp. 1–14). Oxford, UK and New York, NY: Berg.

Aronson, J., & Neysmith, S. (1996). You're not in there to just do the work: Depersonalizing policies and the exploitation of home care workers' labor. *Gender and Society, 10*(1), 59–77.

Ayalon, L. (2009). Family and family-like interactions in households with round-the-clock paid foreign carers in Israel. *Ageing and Society, 29*(5), 671–686.

Aziz, F. (2009). Trends in Labor Force Participation by Race and Gender. Economic School of Business. Hamline University. Available at http://notizie.unimo.it/campusfile/file/atevt/file27790.pdf. Accessed on July 9, 2012.

Azz, M., Cardenas, C., Ciafaloni, F., Franzinetti, V., Osmani, I., & Santi, R. (1998). *Lavoro, genere, etnie*. Quaderni di Ricerca, Turin, Italy: Ires Lucia Morosini.

Bach, J. (2011). Remittances, gender and development. In M. H. Marchand & A. Sisson Runyan (Eds.), *Gender and global restructuring: Sightings, sites, and resistances* (pp. 129–142). New York, NY: Routledge.

Banchero, A., Brizioli, E., & Trabucchi, M. (2013). Reagire alla crisi: come meglio utilizzare le risorse per rispondere ai bisogni delle fragilità. In Network Non Autosufficienza (Ed.), *L'Assistenza agli Anziani Non Autosufficienti in Italia, Tra Crisi e Ripartenza* (pp. 165–184). Santarcangelo di Romagna, Italy: Maggioli Editore.

Barbabella, F., Chiatti, C., Di Rosa, M., & Gori, C. (2013). La bussola di NNA: lo stato dell'arte basato sui dati. In AAVV (Eds.), *L'assistenza agli anziani non autosufficienti in Italia* (pp. 11–28). Santarcangelo di Romagna, Italy: Maggioli editore.

Barbagli, M., Colombo, A., & Sciortino, G. (Eds.). (2004). *I Sommersi e i Sanati. Le regolarizzazioni degli immigrati in Italia.* Bologna, Italia: Il Mulino.

Barbiano di Belgioioso, E., & Ortensi, E. (2013). Should I Stay or Should I Go? The Case of Italy. Rivista Italiana di Economia, Demografia e Statistica, LXVII(3–4), 31–38.

Baumann, G. (1996). *Contesting Culture. Discourses of Identity in Multi-ethnic London.* Cambridge, UK: Cambridge University Press.

Bergqvist, C., & Nyberg, A. (2002). Welfare state restructuring and child care in Sweden. In S. Michel & R. Mahon (Eds.), *Childcare policy at the crossroads. Gender and welfare state restructuring* (pp. 287–309). New York, NY: Routledge.

Bertani, M. (2013). Families in Italy in the face of the crisis of the 'Mediterranean' welfare. *Italian Sociological Review, 3*(2), 85–100.

Bettio, F., & Plantenga, J. (2004). Comparing Care Regimes in Europe. *Feminist Economics, 10*(1), 85–113.

Bettio, F., Simonazzi, A., & Villa, P. (2006). Change in care regimes and female migration: The care drain in the Mediterranean. *Journal of European Social Policy, 16*, 271–285.

Bettio, F., & Verashchagina, A. (2010). Long-term care for the elderly. Provisions and providers in 33 European countries. Report for the European Union. Available at http://ec.europa.eu/justice/gender-equality/files/elderly_care_en.pdf. Accessed February 20, 2013.

Bonanomi, A., Fosti, G., Notarnicola E., & Tasselli, S. (2013). Un welfare che non sa scegliere. *La Voce.* Available at http://www.lavoce.info/un-welfare-che-non-sa-scegliere/#e9WCWGSCwpdYYkBx.99. Accessed June 20, 2013.

Bott, E. (2005). Too close for comfort? Race and the management of proximity, guilt and other anxieties in paid domestic labour. *Sociological Research Online, 10*(3). Available at http://www.socresonline.org.uk/10/3/bott.html. Accessed April 25, 2009.

Bloom, D. E., Boersch-Supan, A., McGee, P., & Atsushi, S. (2011). Population aging: Facts, challenges, and responses. PGDA Working Paper no. 71. Available at http://www.hsph.harvard.edu/pgda/working.html. Accessed September 10, 2011.

Boongarts, J. (2001). The end of the fertility transition in developing countries. Available at: www.un.org/esa/. . ./RevisedBONGAARTSpaper.PDF. Accessed May 20, 2013.

Boongarts, J. (2002). The end of the fertility transition. *Population and Development Review, 28*(3), 419–443.

Boongarts, J. (2009). Human population growth and the demographic transition. *The Philosophical Transactions of the Royal Society of London, Series B, Biological Sciences, 364*(1532), 2985–2990.

Bonizzoni, P. (2013). Undocumented Domestic Workers In Italy: Surviving and Regularizing Strategies. In A. Triandafyllidou (Ed.), *Irregular Domestic Workers in Europe. Who Cares?* (pp. 135–160). Aldershot, UK: Ashgate.

Boris, E., & Parreñas, R. (Eds.) (2010). *Intimate Labors: Cultures, technologies, and the Politics of Care.* Redwood City, CA: Stanford University Press.

Boris, E., & Klein, J. (2012). *Caring for America. Home Health Workers in the Shadow of the Welfare State.* New York, NY and London, UK: Oxford University Press.

Brennan, D., & Williams, F. (2012). Care, markets, and migration in a globalizing world: Introduction to the Special Issue. In *Journal of European Social Policy, 22*(4), 355–362.

Browne, C., & Braun, K. (2008). Globalization, Women's Migration, and the Long-Term-Care Workforce. *The Gerontologist, 48*(1), 16–24.

Bureau of Labor Statistics. (2015a). *Unpaid eldercare in the United States–2013-2014 summary.* Available at http://www.bls.gov/news.release/elcare.nr0.htm. Accessed September 24, 2015.

Bureau of Labor Statistics. (2015b). *Women in the Labor Force: A databook. Report 1059.* Available at http://www.bls.gov/opub/reports/cps/women-in-the-labor-force-a-databook-2015.pdf. Accessed January 3, 2016.

Burgio, A., Battisti, A. Solipaca, A., Colosimo, S.C., Sicuro, L., Damiani, G., Baldassarre, G., Milan, G., Tamburrano, T., Crialesi, E., & Ricciardi, W. (2010). *La Relazione tra Offerta di Servizi di Long-Term Care e i Bisogni Assistenziali dell'Anziano.* Vol. 4. Rome, Italy: ISTAT. Available at http://www3.istat.it/dati/pubbsci/contributi/Contributi/contr_2010/04_2010.pdf. Accessed on October 23, 2013.

Buroway, M. (2000) *Global Ethnography.* Berkeley & Los Angeles: California University Press.

Calavita, K. (2005). *Immigrants at the Margin: Law, Race, and Exclusion in Southern Europe.* Cambridge, UK: Cambridge University Press.

Campani, G. (2004). Italy: Economic Realities, Political Fictions, and Policy Failures. In W. Cornelius, P. L. Martin & J. F. Hollifield (Eds.), *Controlling Immigration: A Global Perspective* (pp. 345–380). Stanford, CA: Stanford University Press.

Campani, G. (2007). Gender and Migration in Italy. State of the Art. Working Paper No. 6 – WP4. Available at www.femipol.uni-frankfurt.de/docs/working_papers/wp3/Italy.pdf. Accessed on March 2, 2014.

Cancedda, A. (2001). *Employment in household services.* Office for Official Publications of the European Communities.

Cangiano, A. (2014). Elder care and migrant labor in Europe: A demographic outlook. *Population and Development Review, 40*(1), 131–154.

Cardenas, C. (1998). *Lavoro, Genere, Etnia.* Turin, Italy: IRES.

CARITAS (2013). Dossier Statistico Immigrazione. *XXIII Rapporto Immigrazione Caritas Migrantes 2013. Tra Crisi e Diritti Umani.* Roma, Italy: IDOS.

Carmichael, F., & Charles, S. (2003). The opportunity costs of informal care: Does gender matter? *Journal of Health Economics, 22*(5), 781–803.

Castells, M. (1996). *The rise of the network society. Vol. 1 of The information age: Economy, society and culture.* Malden, MA: Blackwell.

Castles, S., & Miller, M. J. (2003). *The Age of Migration.* New York, NY: Guilford Press.

Castles, S., de Haas, H., & Miller, M. J. (2013). *The Age of Migration 5th Edition.* New York, NY: Guilford Press.

Catanzaro, R., & Colombo, A. (Eds.) (2009), *Badanti & Co. Il lavoro domestico straniero in Italia.* Bologna, Italy: Il Mulino.

Censis & Fondazione ISMU (2013). *Servizi alla persona e occupazione nel welfare che cambia.* Censis, N.7/8. Available at http://www.censis.it/Censis/browse/28. Accessed on September 28, 2014.

Chang, G. (2000). *Disposable domestics: Immigrant women workers in the global economy.* Boston, MA: South End Press.

Chell-Robinson, V. (2000). Female migrants in Italy: Coping in a country of new migration. In F. Anthias & G. Lazaridis (Eds.), *Gender and migration in Southern Europe: Women on the move* (pp. 103–124). Oxford, UK & New York, NY: Berg.

Clarke, J., Newman, J., Smith, N., Vidler, E., & Westmarland, L. (2007). *Creating Citizen-Consumers: Changing Publics and Changing Public Services.* London, UK: Sage.

Colombo, A. D. (2007). They call me a housekeeper, but I do everything. Who are domestic workers today in Italy and what do they do? *Journal of Modern Italian Studies, 12*(2), 207–237.

Colombo, F. et al. (2011). Help Wanted?: Providing and Paying for Long-Term Care. OECD Health Policy Studies. Paris: OECD.

Cominelli, C. (2003). Filippini nel settore domestico: I limiti di una integrazione subalterna. In M. Ambrosini & F. Berti (Eds.), *Immigrazione e Lavoro.* Milan, Italy: Franco Angeli.

Constable, N. (1997). *Maid to order in Hong Kong: An ethnography of Filipina workers.* Ithaca, NY: Cornell University Press.

Constable, N. (2007). *Maid to order in Hong Kong: Stories of Migrant Workers.* Ithaca, NY, Cornell University Press.

Costa, G. (2013). Long Term Care Italian Policies: A Case of Inertial Institutional Change. In C. Ranci & E. Pavolini (Eds.), *Reforms in Long-Term Policies in Europe* (pp. 221–241). New York, NY: Springer.

Cotesta, V. (2002). *Lo Straniero: Pluralismo culturale e immagini dell'altro nella società globale.* Rome, Italy: Laterza Editori.

Craig, Lyn. (2006). Children and the Revolution. *The Australian Sociological Association*, 42(2), pp.125–143.

Crittenden, Ann. (2001). *The Price of Motherhood.* New York, NY: Metropolitan Books.

Daly, M. (2001). *Care Work. The Quest for Security.* Geneva, Switzerland: International Labor Organization (ILO).

Daly, M., & Lewis, J. (2000). The Concept of Social Care and the Analysis of Contemporary Welfare States. *The British Journal of Sociology, 51*(2), 281–298.

Daly, M., & Standing, G. (2001). Introduction. In Daly, M. (Ed.), *Care Work. The Quest for Security.* Geneva, Switzerland: International Labor Organization (ILO).

Da Roit, B. (2006). La riforma dell'indennità di accompagnamento. In C. Gori (Ed.), *La Riforma dell'Assistenza ai Non Autosufficienti* (pp. 278–315). Bologna, Italy: Il Mulino.

Da Roit, B. (2007). Changing Intergenerational Solidarities within Families in a Mediterranean Welfare State. Elderly Care in Italy. *Current Sociology, 55*(2), 251–269.

Da Roit, B. (2010). *Strategies of care: Changing elderly care in Italy and the Netherlands.* Amsterdam, The Netherlands: Amsterdam University Press.

Da Roit, B., & Facchini, C. (2010). *Anziani e Badanti. Le differenti condizioni di chi è accudito e di chi accudisce.* Milano, Italy: Franco Angeli Editore.

Da Roit B., & Sabatinelli, S. (2005). Il modello mediterraneo di welfare tra famiglia e mercato. *Stato e mercato, 2*, 267–290.

Da Roit, B., & Sabatinelli, S. (2013). Nothing on the move or just going private? Understanding the freeze on child- and eldercare policies and the development of care markets in Italy. *Social Politics, 20*(3), 430–453.

Da Roit, B., & Weicht, B. (2013). Migrant care work and care, migration and employment regimes: A fuzzy-set analysis. *Journal of European Social Policy, 23*(5), 469–486.

Davidson, P., DiGiacomo, M., & McGrath, S. J. (2011). The feminization of aging: How will this impact on health outcomes and services? *Health Care for Women International, 32*(12), 1031–1045.

Degiuli, F. (2007). A job with no boundaries: Home eldercare work in Italy. *European Journal of Women's Studies, 14*(3), 193–207.

Degiuli, F. (2010). The Burden of Long-Term Care: How Italian Family Caregivers Become Employers. *Aging and Society, 30*(5), 755–777.

Degiuli, F. (2011). Laboring Lives: The Making of Home Eldercare Assistants. *Modern Italy. 16*(3), 345–361.

DEMO ISTAT (2013). *Demo-Geodemo. Mappe, Popolazione, Statistiche.* Available at http://demo.istat.it/pop2013/index.html. Accessed on July 20, 2015.

Department of Health and Ageing. (2012). *Living longer. Living better. Aged care reform package* (technical document), April. Commonwealth of Australia, Canberra. Accessed online August 2012. http://www.health.gov.au/internet/publications/publishing.nsf/Content/ageing-living-longer-living-better-reform-package-toc.

Department of Labor (2013) *Minimum wage, overtime protections extended to direct care workers by US Labor Department.* Available at http://www.dol.

gov/whd/media/press/whdpressVB3.asp?pressdoc=national/20130917.xml. Accessed on June 13, 2015.

Deutsch, F. (1999). *Halving it all: How equally shared parenting works.* Cambridge, MA: Harvard University Press.

Dill, B. T. (1994). *Across the boundaries of race and class: An exploration of work and family among black domestic servants.* New York, NY & London, UK: Garland.

Dodson, L., & Zincavage, R. (2007). It's like a family: Caring labor, exploitation, and race in nursing homes. *Gender Society, 21*, 905–929.

Earle, A., & Heymann, J. (2011). Protecting the health of employees caring for family members with special health care needs. *Social Science and Medicine, 173*(1), 66–78.

England, P. (2005). Emerging Theories of Care Work. *Annual Review of Sociology, 31*, 381–399.

Enloe, C. (1989, 2000). *Bananas, Beaches, and Bases: Making Feminist Sense of International Politics.* Los Angeles, CA: California University Press.

Erhenreich, B., & Hochschild, A. (Eds.) (2002). *Global woman: Nannies, maids and sex workers in the new economy.* New York, NY: Owl Books.

Esping-Andersen, G. (1999). *The Social Foundations of Postindustrial Economies.* Oxford, UK: Oxford University Press.

European Commission (2015). *Labour Market Participation of Women.* Available at http://ec.europa.eu/europe2020/pdf/themes/2015/labour_market_participation_of_women.pdf. Accessed January 4, 2016.

Eurostat. (2012a). *Population structure and ageing.* Available at http://epp.eurostat.ec.europa.eu/statistics_explained/index.php/Population structure_and_ageing. Accessed January 2, 2014.

Eurostat. (2012b). *Statistiche dell' occupazione.* Available at http://epp.eurostat.ec.europa.eu/statistics_explained/index.php/Employment_statistics/it. Accessed January 24, 2014.

Eurostat. (2013). *Statistics database*, European Commission. Available at http://epp.eurostat.ec.europa.eu/portal/page/portal/statistics/search_database. Accessed December 10, 2013.

Freeman, C. (2000). *High Tech and High Heels in the Global Economy: Women, Work, and Pink-Collar Identities in the Caribbean.* Durham, NC: Duke University Press.

Foucault, M. (1991). Governmentality. In G. Burchell, C. Gordon & P, Miller (Eds.), *The Foucault Effect: Studies in Governmentality* (pp. 87–104). London, UK: Harvester Wheatsheaf.

Folbre, N. (1983). Of patriarchy born: The political economy of fertility decisions. *Feminist Studies, 9*(2), 261–284.

Folbre, N. (2001). *The Invisible Heart: Economics and Family Values.* New York, NY: New Press.

Fondazione ISMU (2005). *Undicesimo rapporto sulle Migrazioni.* Milano, Italy: Franco Angeli Editore.

Francavilla, F., Giannelli, G. C., Grotkowska, G., & Mieczyslaw, W. S. (2011). Use of time and value of unpaid family care work: A comparison between Italy and Poland. Discussion Paper No. 5771, Forschungsinstitut zur Zukunft der Arbeit (Institute for the Study of Labor). Available at http://ftp.iza.org/dp5771.pdf. Accessed May 14, 2013.

Frontex (2013). *Annual Risk Analysis 2013.* Available at http://frontex.europa.eu/assets/Publications/Risk_Analysis/Annual_Risk_Analysis_2013.pdf. Accessed June 24, 2015.

Fullin, G., & Vercelloni, V. (2009). Dentro la trappola. Percezioni e immagini del lavoro domestic e di cura nei percorsi delle donne immigrate. *Polis*, XXIII(3), 425–461.

Gabaccia, D. (2000). *Italy's Many Diasporas.* London, UK: UCL Press.

Gagliardi, C., Di Rosa, M., Melchiorre, M. G., Spazzafumo, L., & Marcellini, F. (2012). Italy and the Aging Society: Overview of Demographic Trends and Formal/Informal Resources for the Care of Older People. In J. Jaworski (Ed.), *Advances in Sociology Research* (pp. 85–104). Hauppauge, NY: NOVA Publishers.

Galor, O. (2004). The demographic transition and the emergence of sustained economic growth, Working Paper, Brown University, Department of Economics, No.2004-13.

Gamburd, M. R. (2000). *The Kitchen Spoon's Handle.* Ithaca, NY: Cornell University Press.

Gammage, S. (2006). Exporting People and Recruiting Remittances. A Development Strategy for El Salvador?. *Latin American Perspectives*, *33*(6), 75–100.

Giorgi, A. (2012). *The Cultural Construction of Migrant Women in the Italian Press. E-Cadernos, Centro de Estudos Sociais, Universidade de Coimbra.* Available at http://www.ces.uc.pt/e-cadernos/media/ecadernos16/03_Alberta_Giorgi.pdf. Accessed on May 2, 2014.

Glazer, N. Y. (1993). *Women's Paid and Unpaid Labor: The Work Transfer in Health Care and Retailing.* Philadelphia, PA: Temple University Press.

Glendinning, C. (2008). Increasing Choice and Control for Older and Disabled People: A Critical Review of New Developments in England. *Social Policy Administration*, *42*(5), 451–469.

Glenn, E. N. (1992). From Servitude to Service Work: Historical Continuities in the Racial Division of Paid Reproductive Labor. In *Signs*, *18*(1), 1–43.

Glenn, E. N. (2010). *Forced to Care. Coercion and Caregiving in America.* New York, NY: Harvard University Press.

Glucksmann, M., & Lyon, D. (2006). Configurations of care work: Paid and unpaid elder care in Italy and the Netherlands. *Sociological Research Online*, *11*(2).

Goldin, C. (1989). Life-cycle labor-force participation of married women: Historical evidence and implications. *Journal of Labor Economics, 7.1*, 20–47.

Goobermann-Hill, R., & Ebrahim, S. (2006). Informal care at times of change in health and mobility: A qualitative study. *Age and Ageing, 35*(3), 261–266.

Gori, C. (2002). *Il welfare nascosto: il mercato privato dell'assistenza in Italia e in Europa*. Rome, Italy: Carocci Editore.

Gori, C., & Da Roit, B. (2007). The commodification of care – the Italian way. In C. Ungerson, and S. Yeandle (Eds.), *Cash for Care in Developed Welfare States* (pp. 60–80). London, UK: Palgrave.

Gori, C., & Lamura, G. (2009). Lo scenario complessivo. In Network Non Autosufficienza (Eds.), *L'Assistenza agli Anziani Non Autosufficienti in Italia. Rapporto 2009* (pp. 17–34). Santarcangelo di Romagna, Italy: Maggioli Editore.

Gori, C., & Pelliccia, L. (2013). I territori davanti alla crisi. In Network Non Autosufficienza (Eds.), *L'assistenza agli anziani non autosufficienti in Italia*, (pp. 157–182). Roma, Italy: Carrocci Editore.

Gori, C., & Torre, R. (2001). Gli assegni di cura locali. In C. Ranci (Ed.), *L'Assistenza agli Anziani in Italia e in Europa*. Milano, Italy: Franco Angeli Editore.

Gutiérrez Rodriguez, E. (2010). *Migration, Domestic Work and Affect: A Decolonial Approach on Value and the Feminization of Labour*. London, UK: Routledge.

Harper, S. (2005). *Ageing Societies*. London, UK: Routledge.

Harper, S. (2009). Demographic change, generations and the life course. Report for the Ten Challenge Paper, Oxford University. Available at http://www.beyondcurrenthorizons.org.uk/wp-content/uploads/challenge-1-synoptic-report.pdf. Accessed October 28, 2013.

Harper, S., & Leeson, G. (2009). Introducing the journal of population ageing. *Population Ageing*, (2008), *1*, 1–5.

Hayutin, A. (2010). *Population aging will reshape global economics and geopolitics*. Available at longevity3.stanford.edu/wp-content/uploads/2013/01/SCL-Population-Age-Shifts-65+-Handout-May-2010_final-web.pdf. Accessed December 2, 2013.

Heisler, B. S. (1985). Sending countries and the politics of emigration and destination. *In The International Migration Review, 19*(3), 469–484.

Heitmueller, A. (2007). The chicken or the egg?: Endogeneity in labour market participation of informal carers in England. *Journal of Health Economics, 26*(3), 536–559.

Himmelweit, S. (1999). Caring Labor. *The Annals of the American Academy of Political and Social Science, 561*(1), 27–38.

Hochschild, A. (1997). *The time bind: When work becomes home and home becomes work*. New York, NY: Metropolitan Books.

Hochschild, A. (2000). The Nanny Chain. *The American Prospect, 11*(4), 32–36. Available at http://prospect.org/article/nanny-chain. Accessed June 15, 2009.

Hochschild, A. (2003). *The Managed Heart*. Berkeley, CA: University of California Press.

Hondagneu-Sotelo, P. (2001). *Domestica: Immigrant workers cleaning and caring in the shadows of affluence*. Oakland, CA: University of California Press.

Huang, S., & Yeoh, B. S. (2007). Emotional labour and transnational domestic work: the moving geographies of 'maid abuse'in Singapore. *Mobilities, 2*(2), 195–217.

Ibarra, M. (2002). Emotional Proletarian in a Global Economy: Mexican Immigrant Women and Elder Care Work. *Urban Anthropology and Studies of Cultural Systems and World Economic Development, 31*(3/4), 317–350.

Institute for Health Metrics and Evaluation. (2010). *The Global Burden of Disease, Injuries, and Risk Factors Study*. Seattle, WA: IHME. Available at http://www.healthdata.org/gbd. Accessed March 12, 2013.

Institute for Health Metrics and Evaluation. (2013). *The Global Burden of Disease: Generating Evidence, Guiding Policy*. Seattle, WA: IHME. Available at http://www.healthdata.org/policy-report/global-burden-disease-generating-evidence-guiding-policy. Accessed January 6, 2015.

INPS. (Istituto Nazionale di Previdenza Sociale.) (2003). Ricerca Inps-Caritas su immigrazione e collaborazione domestica. Roma, Italy: Caritas.

INPS (2013). *La riforma delle pensioni*. Available at https://www.inps.it/portale/default.aspx?sID=%3B0%3B7661%3B&lastMenu=7661&iMenu=1&p3=2&bi=22&link=La%20riforma%20delle%20pensioni. Accessed January 23, 2014.

ISTAT. (Istituto Nazionale di Statistica). (2003). La vita di coppia. Indagine multiscopo sulle famiglie. Roma: ISTAT.

ISTAT. (2005). *Rapporto Annuale. La situazione del paese nel 2005*. Roma: ISTAT.

ISTAT. (2007). *Annuario Statistico Italiano*. Roma: ISTAT. Available at http://www3.istat.it/dati/catalogo/20071212_00/contenuti.html. Accessed May, 19, 2013.

ISTAT. (2011). *La popolazione straniera residente in Italia*. Available at http://www.west-info.eu/files/RISPOSTAPERCOMUNITASTRANIERA.pdf. Accessed June 21, 2015.

ISTAT. (2013a). *Annuario statistico Italiano*. Roma: ISTAT Available at http://www.istat.it/it/files/2013/12/Cap_2.pdf. Accessed January 2, 2014.

ISTAT. (2013b). *Demografia in cifre*, Roma, Istituto Nazionale di Statistica, www.demo.istat.it. Accessed December 9, 2014.

ISTAT. (2014). *Annuario Statistico*. Available at http://www.istat.it/it/files/2014/11/Asi-2014.pdf. Accessed July 9, 2015.

ISTAT. (2015). *Indicatori Demografici. Stime per l'anno 2014*. Available at https://www.google.com/search?q=ISTAT+indicatore+demografici+2015+tasso+di+dipendenza&ie=utf-8&oe=utf-8. Accessed January 8, 2016.

James, K. S. (2011). India's demographic change: Opportunities and challenges. *Science, 333*, 576–580.

Lloyd, E. (2012) Childcare markets: an introduction. In E. Lloyd and H. Penn (Eds.) *Childcare* markets - *Can they deliver an equitable service?* Bristol, UK: The Policy Press in association with University of Chicago Press.

Lopez, S. H. (2006). Emotional Labor and Organized Emotional Care. Conceptualizing Nursing Home Care Work. *Work & Occupations, 23*(2), 133–160.

Lorente, B. P. (2011). The making of 'Workers of the World.' Language and the labor brokerage state. In A. Duchêne & M. Heller (Eds.), *Language in late capitalism* (pp. 183–206). New York, NY: Routledge.

Lutz, H. (Ed.) (2008). *Migration and domestic work. A European perspective on a global theme.* Aldershot, UK: Ashgate.

Lutz, H. (2011). *The New Maids: Transnational Women and the Care Economy.* London, UK: Zed Books.

Lyon, D. (2006). The organization of care work in Italy: Gender and migrant labor in the new economy. *Indiana Journal of Global Legal Studies, 13*(1), 207–224.

Lyon, D., & Glucksmann, M. 2008. Comparative Configurations of Care Work Across Europe. In *Sociology*, n.42, 101–118.

Mahon, R., & Robinson, F. (Eds.) (2011). *Feminist Ethics and Social Policy. Towards a New Global Political Economy of Care.* Vancouver, CA: UCB Press.

Marchand, M. H., & Runyan, A. S. (Eds.) (2010). *Gender and Global Restructuring: sightings, sites and resistances.* New York, NY: Routledge.

Marchetti, S. (2015). 'Mum Seems Happy'. Relatives of Dependent Elders and the Difficult Task to Employ a Migrant Care-giver. In A. Triandafyllidou & S. Marchetti (Eds.), *Employers, Agencies, and Immigration* (pp. 93–112). Farnham, Surrey: Ashgate.

Martin, C., & Le Bihan, B. (2007). Cash for Care in the French Welfare State: A Skillful Compromise? In Ungerson C, Yeandle S, (Eds.), *Cash for Care Systems in Developed Welfare States* (pp. 32–59). London, UK: Palgrave.

Massey, D. S., Arango, J., Hugo, G., Kouaouci, A., Pellegrino, A., & Taylor, J. E. (1998). *Worlds in motion: Understanding international migration at the end of the millennium.* Oxford, England: Clarendon Press.

Massey, D. S., Durand, J., & Malone, N. J. (2005). Principles of Operation. Theories of International Migration, In C. Suarez Orosco, M. Suarez Orosco & D. Baolian Qin-Hillard (Eds.), *The New Immigration: An Interdisciplinary Reader* (pp. 21–34). New York, NY and London, UK: Routledge.

Mattingly, M. J. & Bianchi, S. M. (2003). Gender Differences in Quantity and Quality of Free Time: The U.S. Experience. *Social Forces*, 81(3), 999–1030.

Mazza, S., & Capacci, G. (2006). L'invecchiamento della popolazione italiana: effetti e politica sociale. *Quaderni Europei sul Nuovo Welfare*, (5). Available at: http://www.newwelfare.org/2006/07/16/l%E2%80%99invecchiamento-della-popolazione-italiana-effetti-e-politica-sociale/. Accessed February 12, 2014.

Mazzacurati, C. (2005). Dal Blat alla vendita di lavoro. Come sono cambiate colf e badanti ucraine e moldave a Padova. In T. Caponio & A. Colombo

(Eds.), *Migrazioni globali, integrazioni locali* (pp. 145–174). Bologna, Italy: Il Mulino.

MacDonald, C. (2011). *Shadow Mothering.* Berkeley, CA: University of California Press.

MacDonald, C., & Sirianni, C. J. (1996). The Service Society and the Changing Experience of Work. In C. MacDonald & C. J. Sirianni (Eds.), *Working in the Service Society* (pp. 1–28). Philadelphia, PA: Temple University Press.

McDonald, Peter. (2000). Gender equity in theories of fertility transition. *Population and Development Review, 26*(3), 427–439.

Merrill, H. (2006). *An Alliance of Women: Immigration and the Politics of Race.* Minneapolis, MN: Minnesota University Press.

Mills, M. B. (1999). *Thai Women in the Global Labor Force: Consuming Desires, Contested Selves.* New Brunswick, NJ: Rutgers University Press.

Ministero del Lavoro e delle Politiche Sociali. (2013). *Rapporto Sulla Coesione Sociale 2013.* Accessible at http://www.west-info.eu/it/come-si-trasforma-la-famiglia-italiana/ministero-del-lavoro-e-delle-politiche-sociali-inps-e-istat-rapporto-sulla-coesione-sociale-anno-2013-i-volume/. Accessed January 1, 2014.

Ministero della Salute (2006). *Piano Sanitario Nazionale 2006 2008.* Available at http://www.salute.gov.it/portale/documentazione/p6_2_2_1.jsp?id=1205. Accessed on April 7, 2007.

Misra, J., Woodring, J., & Merz, S. (2012). The Globalization of Carework: Neoliberal Economic Restructuring and Migration Policy. *Globalization, 3*(3), 317–332.

Murray, M., & Crummett, A. (2010). 'I don't think they knew we could do these sorts of things': Social representations of community and participation in community arts by older people. *Journal of Health Psychology, 15*(5), 777–785.

Naldini, M. (2003). *The Family in the Mediterranean Welfare States.* London, UK: Frank Cass.

Naldini, M., & Saraceno, C. (2008). Social and Family Policies in Italy: Not totally frozen but far from structural reforms. *Social Policy Administration, 42*(7), 733–748.

Naldini, M., & Jurado, T. (2009). The future of the welfare state: paths of social policy innovation between constraints and opportunities. Paper presented at the 7[Th] ESPAnet conference in Urbino. Available at http://www.espanet-italia.net/conference2009/paper2/3-Jurado-Naldini.pdf>. Accessed on May 26, 2013.

Naletto, G. (2014). Le assistenti familiari straniere: il pilastro del nuovo "modello" di welfare. *L'economia dell'Immigrazione, 3*(6). Available at http://www.fondazioneleonemoressa.org/newsite/wp-content/uploads/2014/04/Leconomia-dellimmigrazione-n.-6.pdf. Accessed June 4, 2014.

Näre, L. (2013). Migrancy, Gender and Social Class in Domestic and Social Care Labour in Italy: An Intersectional Analysis of Demand. *Journal of Ethnic and Migration Studies, 39*(4), 601–623.

National Institute for Aging and the National Institutes of Health. (2007). *Why Population Aging Matters: A Global Perspective.* Available at https://www.nia.nih.gov/sites/. . ./WPAM.pdf. Accessed June 1, 2013.

National Institute for Aging and the National Institutes of Health. (2010). *Global health and aging.* Available at http://www.nia.nih.gov/research/publication/global-health-and-aging/preface. Accessed June 10, 2013.

OECD. (1994). *Caring for Frail Elderly People: New Directions in Care.* Paris, France: OECD.

OECD. (2011). *Help wanted. Providing and paying for long-term care.* Geneva, Switzerland: OECD.

OECD. (2016). *OECD.Stat – LFS by Sex and Age Indicators.* Available at https://stats.oecd.org/Index.aspx?DataSetCode=LFS_SEXAGE_I_R#. Accessed on January 4, 2016.

Osservatorio Terza Età/Aging Society. (2006). *Disabili: Quanti sono, con chi vivono e se non ci fosse la famiglia?* Available at http://www.ageingsociety.com/index.asp?view=studi. Retrieved April 15, 2007.

Österle, A., & Hammer, E. (2007). Care Allowances and the Formalization of Care Arrangements: The Austrian Experience. In: Ungerson C, Yeandle S (Eds.), *Cash for Care Systems in Developed Welfare States* (pp. 13–31). London, UK: Palgrave; 2007.

Padavic, I., & Reskin, B. (2002). *Women and Men at Work.* 2nd edition. Washington, D.C.: Sage.

Pagliai, V. (2013). Politics, Citizenship and the Construction of Immigrant Communities in Italy. In P. Kretsedemas, J. Capetillo-Ponce & G. Jacobs (Eds.), *Migrant Marginality: A Transnational Perspective* (pp. 47–62).

Palese, A., Oliverio, F., Girardo, M. F., Fabbro, E., & Saiani, L. (2004). Difficulties and workload of foreign caregivers: A descriptive analysis. *Diversity in Health and Social Care, 1*, 31–38.

Parks, J. A. (2003). *No place like home?: Feminist ethics and home health care.* Indiana University Press. Bloomington, IN: Indiana University Press.

Parreñas, R. S. (2001). *Servants of globalization: Women, migration, and domestic work.* Stanford, CA: Stanford University Press.

Parreñas, R. S. (2006). Migrant Filipina Domestic Workers and International Division of Reproductive Labor. In M. K. Zimmerman, J. S. Litt & C. E. Bose (Eds.), Global Dimensions of Gender and Carework. Stanford, California: Stanford University Press.

Parreñas, R. S. (2014). Migrant Domestic Workers as 'One of the Family.' In B. Anderson & I. Shutes (Eds.), *Migration and Care Labour* (pp. 49–64). London, UK: Palgrave Macmillan.

Pasquinelli, S., & Rusmini, G. (2013). *Badare non basta. Il lavoro di cura: attori, progetti, politiche.* Roma, Italy: Ediesse.

Pavolini, E., & Ranci, C. (2008). Restructuring the Welfare State: Reforms in Long-term Care in Western European countries. *Journal of European Social Policy, 18*(3), 246–259.

Pavolini, E., & Ranci, C. (Eds.) (2013). *Reforms in Long-Term Care Policies in Europe.* New York, NY: Springer.

Piazza, M. (1997). L'ostinata permanenza della non-ovvietà. *Quaderni di Azione Sociale, 1,* 79–86.

Pickard, L. (2011). The supply of informal care in Europe. ENEPRI Research Report No. 94, CEPS, Brussels. Available at http://www.ancien-longtermcare.eu/sites/default/files/ENEPRI%20RR94%20_ANCIEN%20WP%203_%20Supply%20of%20Informal%20Care%20in%20Europe_0.pdf. Accessed March 27, 2013.

Pesaresi, F., & Gori, C. (2005). L'Assistenza agli Anziani Non Autosufficienti in Europa. In C. Facchini (Ed.), *Anziani e Sistemi di Welfare. Lombardia, Italia, Europa.* Milano, Italy: Franco Angeli Editore.

Piore, M. J. (1979). *Birds of Passage. Migrant Labor and Industrial Societies.* Cambridge, UK: Cambridge University Press.

Pojmann, W. (2006). *Immigrant women and feminism in Italy.* Burlington, VT: Ashgate.

Polverini, F., Principi, A., Balducci, C., Melchiorre, M. G., Quattrini, S., Gianelli, M. V., & Lamura, G. (2004). *National Background Report for Italy,* EUROFAMCARE; Available at www.uke.uni-hamburg.de/extern/eurofamcare/documents/nabare_ italy_rc1_a5.pdf. Accessed March 8, 2006.

Portes, A. (1997). Neoliberalism and the Sociology of Development: Emerging Trends and Unanticipated Facts. In *Population and Development Review, 23*(2), 229–259.

Pugliese, E. (2002). *L'Italia tra Migrazioni Internazionali e Migrazioni Interne.* Bologna, Italy: Il Mulino.

Pyle, J., & Ward, K. (2003). Recasting our understanding of gender and work during global restructuring. *International Sociology, 18*(3), 461–489.

Rabiee, P. (2013) Exploring the relationships between choice and independence: experiences of disabled and older people. *British Journal of Social Work, 43*(5), 872–888.

Radin, M. (1996). *Contested Commodities.* Harvard, MA: Harvard University Press.

Ranci, C. (2001). Verso un mercato sociale dei servizi di cura. Prospettive per le politiche assistenziali rivolte alla popolazione anziana. In C. Ranci (Ed.), *L'assistenza agli anziani in Italia e in Europa* (pp. 1–15). Milan, Italy: Franco Angeli Editore.

Ranci, C. (2002). Il welfare sommerso delle badanti. www.lavoce.it. Article appeared on December 2, 2002.

Ranci, C., & Sabatinelli, S. (2014). Long-term and Child Care Policies in Italy between Familism and Privatisation. In Leon, M. (Ed.), *The Transformation of Care in European Societies* (pp. 233–255). London, UK: Palgrave Macmillan.

Reher, D. S. (2011). Economic and social implications of the demographic transition. *Population and Development Review, 37,* 11–33.

Reher, D. (2012). Population and the economy during the demographic transition. *Economic Affairs, 32*(1), 10–16.

Reichstadt, J., Sengupta, G., Depp, C., Palinkas, L., & Jeste, D. (2010). Older adults' perspectives on successful aging qualitative interviews. *American Journal of Geriatric Psychiatry, 18*(7), 567–575. doi:U103.02.04.102.

Reyneri, E. (2001). *Migrants' Involvement in Irregular Employment in the Mediterranean Countries of the European Union.* Geneva, CH: ILO.

Reyneri, E. (2011). *Sociologia del Mercato del Lavoro. Vol. II. Le Forme di Occupazione.* Bologna, Italy: Il Mulino.

Riley, J. C. (2001). *Rising life expectancy: A global history.* Cambridge, UK, Cambridge University Press.

Riley, J. C. (2005). Estimates of global and regional life expectancy, 1800–2001. *Population and Development Review, 31*(3), 537–543.

Rizza, R., & Santangelo, F. (2014). Scelte occupazionali e regolazione: Il lavoro di cura delle donne fra bambini e anziani. *Sociologia del Lavoro, 135*(3), 126–141.

Roberts, D. E. (1997). Spiritual and Menial Housework. *Yale JL & Feminism,* 9(51), 51–80.

Robinson, W. I. (2007). Theories of globalization. In G. Ritzer (Ed.), *The Blackwell Companion to Globalization* (pp. 125–143). Malden, MA: Blackwell Publishing.

Robinson, W. I. (2009). Saskia Sassen and the Sociology of Globalization: A Critical Appraisal. *Sociological Analysis, 3*(1), 5–29.

Rodriguez, J. (2011) 'It's a Dignity Thing': Nursing Home Care Workers' Use of Emotions. *Sociological Forum, 26*(2), 265–286.

Rodriguez, R. M. (2010). *Migrants for export: How the Philippine state brokers labor to the world.* Minneapolis, MN: U of Minnesota Press.

Rollins, J. (1985). *Between women. Domestics and their employers.* Philadelphia, PA: Temple University Press.

Romero, M. (1992). *Maid in the U.S.A.* New York, NY & London, UK: Routledge.

Romero, M. (2002). *Maid in the U.S.A. Tenth Anniversary Edition.* New York, NY & London, UK: Routledge.

Sadasivam, B. (1997). The impact of structural adjustment on women: A governance and human rights agenda. *Human Rights Quarterly, 19*(3), 630–665.

Sabbadini, L. (2002). La rete di aiuti informali. Osservatorio nazionale sulle famiglie e le politiche locali di sostegno alle responsabilità familiari. *Famiglie: mutamenti e politiche sociali,* vol. II. 329–356.

Salomon, J. A., Wang, H., Freeman, M. K., Vos, T., Flaxman, A. D., Lopez, A. D., et al. (2012). Healthy life expectancy for 187 countries, 1990–2010: a systematic analysis for the Global Burden Disease Study 2010. *Lancet, 380*(9859), 2144–2162.

Saltman, R. B., Rico, A., & Boerma, W. (2006). *Primary care in the driver's seat? Organizational reform in European primary care.* Maidenhead, UK: Open University Press.

Saraceno, C. (2003a). La conciliazione di responsabilità familiari e attività lavorative in Italia: paradossi ed equilibri imperfetti. *Polis,* (2), 199–228.

Saraceno, C. (2003b). *Mutamenti della Famiglia e Politiche Sociali in Italia.* Bologna, Italy: Il Mulino.

Sarti, R. (2004). Noi abbiamo visto tante città, abbiamo un'altra cultura. Servizio domestico, migrazioni e identità di genere in Italia: uno sguardo di lungo periodo. *Polis, 1,* 17–46.

Sarti, R. (2008). The Globalisation of Domestic Service in a Historical Perspective. In H. Lutz (Ed.), *Migration and Domestic Work: A European Perspective on a Global Theme* (pp. 77–98). Aldershot, UK: Ashgate.

Sarti, R. (2013). Italia domestica. Breve storia del personale di servizio. In S. Pasquinelli & G. Rusmini (Eds.), *Badare non basta. Il lavoro di cura: attori, progetti, politiche* (pp. 19–40). Roma, Italy: Ediesse, 2013.

Sassen, S. (1988). *The Mobility of Capital and Labor: A Study in International Investment and Labor Flow.* Cambridge, UK: Cambridge University Press.

Sassen, S. (1984). Notes on the Incorporation of Third World Women into Wage Labor through Immigration and Offshore Production. *International Migration Review, 18,* 1144–1167.

Sassen, S. (1999). *Globalization and its Discontents: Essays on the New Mobility of People and Money.* New York, NY: New Press

Sassen, S. (1991, 2001). *The Global City: New York, London, Tokyo.* Princeton, NJ: Princeton University Press.

Schierup, C. U., Hansen, P., & Castles, S. (2006). Economic Miracle and Political Limbo: Italy and its 'Extracommunitarians.' In C.U. Schierup, P. Hansen, S. Castles (Eds.), *Migration, Citizenship, and the Italian Welfare State* (pp. 163–194). Oxford, UK: Oxford University Press.

Scrinzi, F. (2004). Professioniste della tradizione. Le donne migranti nel mercato del lavoro domestico. *Polis, 1,* 107–136.

Sgritta, G. B. (2009). *Badanti e Anziani: In un welfare senza future.* Rome, Italy: Edizioni Lavoro.

Shutes, I., & Chiatti, C. (2012). Migrant labour and the marketisation of care for older people: The employment of migrant care workers by families and service providers. *Journal of European Social Policy, 22*(4), 392–405.

Silverstein, M., & Giarrusso, R. (2010). Aging and Family Life: A Decade Review. *Journal of Marriage and Family, 72*(5), 1039–1058.

Simmel, G. (1908/1971). *On individuality and social forms.* Chicago, IL: University of Chicago Press.

Simonazzi, A. (2009). Care regimes and national employment models. *Cambridge Journal of Economics, 33*(2), 211–232.

Sirkeci, I., Cohen, J. H., & Ratha, D. (Eds.) (2012). *Migration and Remittances during the Global Financial Crisis and Beyond.* Washington, DC.: The World Bank.

Smiley, S. (2013). Observations on Aging and Eldercare in Japan. *Journal of Aging in Emerging Economies, 4*(1), 35–59.

Solari, C. (2011). Between Europe and Africa: Building the New Ukraine on the shoulders of migrant women. In M. J. Rubchak (Ed.), *Mapping difference: The many faces of women in Ukraine* (pp. 23–40). New York, NY & Oxford, UK: Berghahn Books.

Solari, C. (2014). Gendered global ethnography. Comparing migration patterns and Ukrainian emigration. In P. Kretsedemas, J. Capetillo-Ponce, & G. Jacobs (Eds.), *Migrant marginality. A transnational perspective.* New York, NY: Routledge.

Spano, P. (2006). *Le convenienze nascoste. Il fenomeno badanti e le risposte del welfare.* Portogruaro (Venice), Italy: Nuova Dimensione.

Stacey, C. (2005). Finding Dignity in Dirty Work: The Constraints and Rewards of Low-Wage Home Care Labor. *Sociology of Health and Illness, 27*(6), 831–854.

Stacey, C. (2011). *The caring self: The work experiences of home care aides.* Ithaca, NY: ILR/Cornell University Press.

Standing, G. (1999). *Global labour flexibility*. Basingstoke, UK: Macmillan.

Stone, R. (2011). *Long-Term Care for the Elderly.* Washington, D.C.: Urban Institute Press.

Taguieff, P.-A. (2001). *The force of prejudice: On racism and its double.* Minneapolis, MN: University of Minnesota Press.

Theobald, S., & Hampel, S. (2013). Radical Institutional Change and Incremental Transformation. In C. Ranci and E. Pavolini (Eds.), *Reform in Long-Term Care Policies in European Countries* (pp. 117–138). Heidelberg and New York: Springer.

Timonen, V. (2008). *Ageing societies: A comparative introduction.* Maidenhead, UK: Open University Press.

Tognetti Bordogna, M. (2012). *Donne e percorsi migratori. Per una sociologia delle migrazioni. Milano*, Italy: Franco Angeli.

Troisi, J. (2013). Demographic outlook of ageing in the Mediterranean, 1950–2050. In J. Troisi & H. J. Von Kondratowitz (Eds.), *Ageing in the Mediterranean.* Bristol, UK: Policy Press.

Triandafyllidou, A., & Marchetti, S. (2015). The Employers' Perspective on Paid Domestic and Care Work. In A. Triandafyllidou & S. Marchetti (Eds.), *Employers, Agencies, and Immigration. Paying for Care* (pp. 1–16). Farnham, UK: Ashgate.

Tsing, A. L. (2005). *Friction: An Ethnography of Global Connection.* Princeton, NJ: Princeton University Press.

Unger, J. B., Ander Johnson, C., & Marks, G. (1997). Functional Decline in the Elderly: Evidence for Direct and Stress-Buffering Protective Effects of Social Interactions and Physical Activity. *Analysis of Behavioral Medicine, 19*(2), 152–160.

Ungerson, C. (2000). Cash in care. In M. Harrington-Meyer (Ed.), *Care work: Gender, class, and the welfare state* (pp. 68–88). New York, NY: Routledge.

Ungerson, C., & Yeandle, S. (2007). *Cash for Care in Developed Welfare States.* London, UK: Palgrave Macmillan.

Unipol-Censis (2014). *Integrare il welfare, sviluppare la white economy.* Roma, Italy, Censis. Available at http://www.regioni.it/sociale/2014/07/09/censis-unipol-rapporto-2014-welfare-italia-laboratorio-per-le-nuove-politiche-sociali-09-07-2014-356234/. Accessed on May 9, 2015.

United Nations Department of Economic and Social Affairs, Popoulation Division (2010a). Population Facts. Available at http://www.un.org/en/development/desa/population/publications/pdf/popfacts/popfacts3.pdf. Accessed April 4, 2013.

United Nations Department of Economic and Social Affairs, Population Division. (2010b). *World population chart.* Available at www.un.org/en/development/desa/population/publications/pdf/trends/WPP2010/WPP2010_Wallchart.pdf. Accessed October 22, 2013.

United Nations Department of Economic and Social Affairs, Population Division. (2012). *The age and sex of migrants.* Available at http://www.un.org/en/development/desa/population/publications/pdf/migration/age-sex-migrants-wallchart_2011.pdf. Accessed June 24, 2013.

United Nations Department of Economic and Social Affairs, Population Division (2013a). *International Migration Report.* New York: United Nations. Available at http://www.un.org/en/development/desa/population/publications/pdf/migration/migrationreport2013/Full_Document_final.pdf. Accessed September 27, 2015.

United Nations Department of Economic and Social Affairs, Population Division (2013b). *World Population Prospects: The 2012 Revision, Methodology of the United Nations Population Estimates and Projections.* Working Paper No. ESA/P/WP.235. New York: United Nations. Available at http://www.un.org/en/development/desa/population/publications/pdf/fertility/Fertility-levels-and-trends_WPP2012.pdf. Accessed January 6, 2016.

United Nations Population Division. (2011). *World population prospects: The 2010 revision.* New York, NY: UN Population Division.

United Nations Population Division. (2012a). *Population ageing and development.* New York, NY: UN Population Division. Available at http://www.un.org/esa/population/publications/2012PopAgeingDev_Chart/2012PopAgeingandDev_WallChart.pdf. Accessed October 10, 2013.

United Nations Population Division. (2012b). Towards global equity in longevity. *Population Facts, 2*, 1–4.

United Nations Department of Economic and Social Affairs, Population Division. (2013). *World population ageing 2013*. New York, NY: UNPD. Available at http://www.un.org/en/development/desa/population/publications/pdf/ageing/WorldPopulationAgeing2013.pdf. Accessed October 15, 2013.

United Nations Population Fund. (2012). *Ageing in the 21st century: A celebration and a challenge*. New York, NY: UNFPA. Available at http://www.unfpa.org/sites/default/files/pubpdf/Ageing%20report.pdf. Accessed October 10, 2013.

US Department of Health and Human Services. (2015). *Who needs care?* http://longtermcare.gov/the-basics/who-needs-care/. Accessed June 15, 2015.

Van de Kaa, D. J. (1987). Europe's second demographic transition. *Population Bulletin, 42* (1). Washington, DC: The Population Reference Bureau.

van Hooren, F. (2011). *Caring migrants in European welfare regimes. The policies and practice of migrant labour filling the gaps in social care*. PhD Dissertation. Florence: European University Institute.

Van Hooren, F. (2012). Varieties of migrant care work, comparing patterns of migrant labour in social care. *Journal of European Social Policy, 22*(2), 133–147.

van Hooren, F. (2014). *Migrant care work in Europe: Variety and institutional determinants*. London, UK: Palgrave Macmillan.

Vega Solis, C. (2009). *Culturas del Cuidadoen Transiciòn*. Barcelona, Spain: Editorial UOC, Niberta.

Viitanen, T. K. (2005). Cost of childcare and female employment in the UK. *Labour, 19*(1), 149–170.

Vietti, F. (2012). *Il Paese delle Badanti*. Turin, Italy: SEI.

Wiles, J., Leibing, A., Guberman, N., Reeve, J., & Allen, R. (2011). The Meaning of "Aging in Place" to Older People. *The Gerontologist, 52*(3), 357–366.

Williams, F. (2005). A good enough life: Developing a political ethic of care. *Surroundings: A Journal of Politics and Culture, 30*(Summer 2005), 17–32.

Williams, F. (2011). Towards A Transnational Analysis of the Political Economy of Care. In Mahon, R. & Robinson, F. (Eds.), *Feminist Ethics and Social Policy. Towards a New Global Political Economy of Care* (pp. 21–38). Vancouver, CA: UCB Press.

Williams, F. (2012). Converging Variations in Migrant Care Work in Europe. *Journal of European Social Policy, 22*(4), 363–376.

Williams, F., & Gavanas, A. (2008). The intersection of child care regimes and migration regimes: A three-country study. In H. Lutz (Ed.), *Migration and domestic work: A European perspective on a global theme*. London, UK: Routledge.

World Bank. (2014). *Data bank: Fertility rate, total (births per woman)*. Available at http://data.worldbank.org/indicator/SP.DYN.TFRT.IN. Accessed October 22, 2013.

World Bank. (2015). *Population estimates and projections*. Available at http://data.worldbank.org/data-catalog/population-projection-tables. Accessed July 6, 2015.

World Health Organization (2010) World Statistics. Available at http://www.who.int/gho/publications/world_health_statistics/EN_WHS10_Full.pdf. Accessed August 25, 2013.

World Health Organization. (2012a). Global Health Observatory: Life expectancy. Available at http://www.who.int/gho/mortality_burden_disease/life_tables/situation_trends_text/en/index.html. Accessed February 22, 2013.

World Health Organization. (2012b). Why focusing on ageing and health, now? World Health Organization Factsheet available at http://www.emro.who.int/world-health-days/2012/fact-sheets.html. Accessed online October 3, 2012.

Wrigley, J. (1995). *Other people's children*. New York, NY: Basic Books.

Yeates, N. (2009). *Globalising care economies and migrant workers: explorations in global care chains*. London, UK: Palgrave.

Zanatta, A. L. (2005). Lavoro di Cura, Genere e Migrazioni. In *Famiglie e Politiche di Welfare in Italia: Interventi e Pratiche* (pp. 50–72). Bologna, Italy: IL Mulino.

Zlotnik, H. (2003). The Global Dimension of Female Migration. Migration Information Source. Available at http://www.migrationpolicy.org/article/global-dimensions-female-migration. Accessed on Feb 10, 2012.

Zontini, E. (2002). Female Domestic Labour Migrants and Local Policies in Bologna: The Story of a Filipino Woman. In R. Grillo & J. Pratt (Eds.), *The Politics of Recognizing difference: Multi-Culturalism Italian Style* (pp. 159–176). Burlington, VT: Ashgate Publications.

Zucchetti, E. (Ed.) (2004). *La Regolarizzazione degli Stranieri. Nuovi attori nel mercato del lavoro italiano*. Milano, Italy: Franco Angeli Editore.

Kaufman, G. (2000). Do gender role attitudes matter? *Journal of Family Issues, 21*(1), 128–144.

Kilkey, M., Lutz, H., & Palenga-Möllenbeck, E. (2010). Introduction: Domestic and Care Work at the Intersection of Welfare, Gender and Migration Regimes: European Experiences. *Social Policy and Society, 9*(3), 379–384.

Kilkey, M., Perrons, D., & Plomien, A. (2013). *Gender, migration and domestic work: Masculinities, male labour and fathering in the UK and USA. Migration, diaspora and citizenship.* London, UK: Palgrave Macmillan Publishers.

Kim, K., & Antonopolous, R. (2011). Unpaid and paid care: The effects of child care and elder care on the standard of living. Working paper no. 691. Levy Economic Institute of Bard College. Available at http://www.levyinstitute.org/pubs/wp_691.pdf. Accessed February 10, 2013.

Kofman, E., Phizacklea, A., Raghuram, P., & Sales, R. (2000). *Gender and International Migration in Europe: employment, welfare, and politics.* London, UK: Routledge.

Kofman, E. (2012). Rethinking care through social reproduction: articulating circuits of migration. *Social Politics, 19*(1), 142–162.

Knijn, T. (2001). Care Work: Innovations in the Netherlands. In M. Daly (Ed.), *Care Work. The Quest for Security* (pp. 159–174). Geneva, Switzerland: International Labor Organization (ILO).

Kunz, R. (2011). *The political economy of global remittances: Gender and governmentality.* New York, NY: Routledge.

Lan, P.-C. (2006). *Global cinderellas: Migrant domestics and newly rich employers in Taiwan.* Durham, NC: Duke University Press.

Lee, R. (2003). The demographic transition: Three centuries of fundamental change. *Journal of Economic Perspectives, 17*(4), 167–190.

Lee, R. (2011). The outlook for population growth. *Science, 333*(6042), 569–573.

Lee, R. D., & Reher, D. S. (2011). Introduction: The landscape of demographic transition and its aftermath. *Population and Development Review, 37*(1), 1–7.

Lister, R. Williams, F., Anttonen, A., Bussemaker, J., Gerhard, U, Heinen, J, Johansson, S., Leira, A., Siim, B., Tobio, C., & Gavanas, A. (2007). *Gendering Citizenship in Western Europe, New Challenges for Citizenship Research in a Crossnational Context.* Bristol, UK: The Policy Press.

Lindio-McGovern, L. (2012). *Globalization, labor export and resistance: A study of Filipino migrant domestic workers in global cities.* New York, NY: Routledge.

Lippi Bruno, M. & Ugolino, C. (2013). *Delegating home care for the elderly to external caregivers? An empirical study on Italian data.* Working Papers wp905, Dipartimento Scienze Economiche, Universita' di Bologna. Available at https://ideas.repec.org/f/c/psi628.html. Accessed on Jan, 29, 2014.

Lloyd, E. (2010). Comparing childcare market developments in England and the Netherlands. Social Policy Association Conference, Lincoln University, 5–7 July.

INDEX

Note: Page numbers followed by *f* indicate a figures; and *t* indicate a tables.